AF682252

The American Civil War Surgery Series

Edited by Ira M. Rutkow, M.D., Dr.P.H.

1. S. D. Gross: *A Manual of Military Surgery* (Philadelphia, 1861)

2. S. P. Moore: *A Manual of Military Surgery, Prepared for the Use of the Confederate States Army*. (Richmond, 1863)

3. S. W. Mitchell, G. R. Morehouse and W. W. Keen: *Gunshot Wounds and Other Injuries of Nerves* (Philadelphia, 1864)

4. J. J. Chisolm: *A Manual of Military Surgery* (Richmond, 1861)

5. F. H. Hamilton: *A Practical Treatise on Military Surgery* (New York, 1861)

6. E. Warren: *An Epitome of Practical Surgery for Field and Hospital* (Richmond, 1863)

7. C. S. Tripler and G. C. Blackman: *Hand-book for the Military Surgeon* (Cincinnati, 1861)

8. S. Smith: *Hand-book of Surgical Operations* (New York, 1862)

9. F. Formento: *Notes and Observations on Army Surgery* (New Orleans, 1863), bound with:

   M. Schuppert: *A Treatise on Gun-shot Wounds: Written for and Dedicated to the Surgeons of the Confederate States Army* (New Orleans, 1861)

10. J. H. Packard: *A Manual of Minor Surgery* (Philadelphia, 1863)

11. Adjutant-General and the Surgeon-General: *List of Battles and Roster of Regimental Surgeons and Assistant Surgeons During the War of the Rebellion* (Washington, D.C., 1883)

NOTES AND OBSERVATIONS ON ARMY SURGERY

and

A TREATISE ON GUN-SHOT WOUNDS

NOTES AND OBSERVATIONS ON ARMY SURGERY

by Felix Formento, Jr., M.D.

bound with

A TREATISE ON GUN-SHOT WOUNDS:

Written for and Dedicated to the Surgeons of the Confederate States Army

by Moritz Schuppert, M.D.

Reprinted with Biographical Introductions

by Ira M. Rutkow, M.D., Dr.P.H.

Norman Publishing
San Francisco
1990

Copyright © 1990 by Norman Publishing

Published by Norman Publishing
Division of Jeremy Norman & Co., Inc.
442 Post Street
San Francisco, California 94102–1579

All rights reserved. No part of this publication may be reproduced, stored in a retrieval system, or transmitted, in any form or by any means, electronic, mechanical, photocopying, recording, or otherwise, without the prior written permission of the publisher, except in the case of brief quotations embodied in critical articles and reviews.

Library of Congress Cataloging-in-Publication Data

Formento, Felix, 1837–1907.
Notes and observations on army surgery / by Felix Formento. Bound with A treatise on gun-shot wounds / written for and dedicated to the surgeons of the Confederate States Army by Moritz Schuppert ; reprinted with biographical introductions by Ira M. Rutkow.
p. cm. — (The American Civil War surgery series ; no. 9)
Reprint (1st work). Originally published: New Orleans : L. E. Marchand, Printer, 1863.
Reprint (2nd work). Originally published: New Orleans : Printed at the Bulletin Book and Job Office, 1861.
ISBN 0–930405–18–8 (alk. paper)
1. Surgery, Military. 2. Gunshot wounds—Treatment.

I. Schuppert, Moritz, 1817–1887. Treatise on gun-shot wounds. 1990. II. Title, III. Series.
RD151.F65 1990
617'.99 — dc19

The American Civil War Surgery Series, No. 9

This volume was reproduced from original editions loaned from the Louisiana Collection, Howard-Tilton Memorial Library, Tulane University.

This book is printed on acid-free paper, and its binding materials have been chosen for strength and durability.

Manufactured in the United States of America.

NOTES AND OBSERVATIONS ON ARMY SURGERY

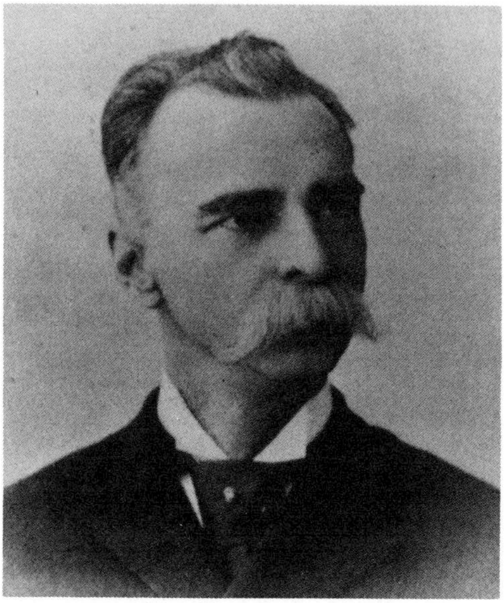

Felix Formento, Jr.

1837–1907

Portrait Collection, Rudolph Matas Medical Library

Tulane University

Felix Formento, Jr.

Born in New Orleans on March 16, 1837, Felix Formento, Jr., was the son of Felix Formento, Sr. (1790–1888) and Palmyra Lauve. His father was a physician, and Felix Jr. followed in his father's footsteps. He received his early education at Jefferson College in his native city but in 1851 his father decided to move the entire family to Italy. Like his father, Felix Jr. matriculated at the Royal University of Turin and in July 1857 obtained his medical degree. Following graduation he studied with his father and eventually went to Paris, where he attended a semester of medical lectures.

Formento practiced for a few months in both Paris and Nice. When France and Sardinia declared war against Austria in 1859, his father asked him to return to Turin to begin his medical career on the battlefield. Consequently, the younger Formento joined the Franco-Sardinian army under the command of Napoleon III. Formento took an active part in the short Italian campaign of 1859. Assigned to the staff of the Third Division under Generals Durando and Mollard, he saw action at Magenta and Solferino.

In the spring of 1860, the elder Formento decided to return to the United States. His son travelled with him and became a visiting surgeon to the Charity Hospital. With the outbreak of the Civil War, Formento was appointed under the auspices of the Louisiana Soldiers' Relief Association to go to Missouri and establish a hospital for the aid of Louisiana soldiers serving in that state. However, Missouri was soon abandoned by the Confederacy and the project was never carried out.

Formento turned his attention to Virginia. Following the heavy fighting around Richmond in July 1861, he established another Louisiana Relief Organization and by October had opened a 300-bed hospital for enlisted men as well as a smaller one for officers. Formento continued as chief surgeon to the Louisiana Hospital through September 1864, when he was forced to resign because of his own poor health and that of his new wife.

In 1863 Formento published *Notes and Observations on Army Surgery*, which was based on his experiences at the Louisiana Hospital in Richmond. This treatise shows that Formento was a sound medical observer and possessed common sense. The mortality rate at the Louisana Hospital was much lower than that in regular army hospitals, and this was attributed to the use of women nurses, small wards, cleanliness, good food, and ample fresh air provided by canvas tent walls that could be lifted up. Formento insisted that penetrating wounds of the abdomen never be probed and that as a general rule trephining should be avoided. His wisdom concerning erysipelas and hospital gangrene was evident in his assertion that any patient showing symptoms of these diseases should be isolated and strict hygiene enforced. It is unclear whether Formento's book was widely circulated and to what extent his ideas were employed.

On resigning his commission, Formento had intended to travel to Europe and meet his father (who had left New Orleans in 1862 after the fall of that city). Unfortunately, his financial affairs were in such a poor state that he had little choice but to stay in the United States and resume the private practice of medicine in New Orleans.

After returning to New Orleans, Formento became associated with James Trudeau (1817–1887) and spent most of his time managing the Baronne Street and Circus Street infirmaries. He was also appointed successively physician of the Italian, the New Lusitanos, the Old Portuguese, and the Firemen's Charitable Associations. He performed his best-known clinical work in connection with New Orleans' yellow fever epidemics of 1867 and 1878. In recognition of his dedication to the Italian citizens of the city, the Italian government bestowed upon him the order of St. Mauritius and Lazarus.

Most of Formento's later years were spent studying epidemiology and infectious diseases. In March 1880, he was appointed by the governor to the Louisiana State Board of Health. He served a full four-year term but lost in an election of the board members in 1884 to succeed Joseph Jones (1833–1896) as president of the board. Formento was disturbed by the loss of this election because he was the senior medical member of the board. As a result, he resigned his position with the statement that evidently his services had not been appreciated.

Among the many advances that Formento had introduced while serving on the State Board of Health were the flushing of streets, creation of a chemical laboratory for the board's use, and a diphtheria registration for physicians. He had also been the major force in creating a spirit of conciliation and cooperation with sanitary organizations in Louisiana and bordering states. Because of his endeavors, the board appointed him as a delegate to the Fourth International Congress of Hygiene and Demography, held in Geneva in September 1882.

In 1886 Formento served as president of the New Orleans Parish Medical Society. The following year he was named secretary of the section on hygiene of the International Medical Congress in Washington. In 1890 the governor reappointed Formento to the State Board of Health, and he served another four-year term. His prominence in the field of public health continued to grow, and as a result Formento was elected president of the American Public Health Association in 1892. He later founded the first cremation society in New Orleans.

Formento performed several notable surgical operations. Among these were a successful removal of the entire elbow joint in the left arm of a Confederate soldier, one of the earliest, albeit unsuccessful, cesarean sections in New Orleans, and the cosmetic repair of the face of a young woman. He was also the first surgeon in New Orleans to utilize plaster of paris as a body cast to treat deformities of the spine.

Formento's first marriage was in 1861 to Celestine Voorhies, who died in 1875 in Nice; she left one son, William J. Formento, who later became an attorney. Formento married Louise Chiapella in 1878. He died in New Orleans from heart disease on June 4, 1907.

NOTES

AND

OBSERVATIONS

—ON—

Army Surgery,

BY

Dr. F. FORMENTO Jr.,

SURGEON IN THE FRANCO-SARDINIAN ARMY

DURING THE ITALIAN CAMPAIGN OF 1859;

LATE CHIEF SURGEON OF THE LOUISIANA HOSPITAL

OF RICHMOND, etc.

NEW ORLEANS.

1863.

L. E. MARCHAND, PRINTER, 201, CHARTRES STREET,

BETWEEN MAIN AND ST. ANN.

PREFACE.

This work is the result of two years' experience at the head of a large military hospital. It is purely professional and written in a practical point of view. Army practice is extensive and infinitely varied; every possible case of diseases and wounds comes under the treatment of the military surgeon. It would be hardly possible, therefore, that some of the remarks in the following pages should not be found worthy of the attention of the general practitioner. They also relate to circumstances and incidents that can scarcely fail to interest the whole public. Nor is it necessary to say that most of the deductions from military practice and experience herein recorded, apply not less to the treatment of ordinary cases of wounds and diseases.

Modestly hoping that the work may contribute in some degree to relieve suffering and save human life, the author submits it to the public consideration.

NEW ORLEANS, November 10th, 1863.

NOTES AND OBSERVATIONS

— ON —

Army Surgery,

BY DR. F. FORMENTO JR,

War seems to be a social necessity. It is in human nature. It has existed ever since the beginning of Creation and will probably continue to exist as long as there are men, — consequently passions, errors and prejudices.— In spite of all the reasoning of philosophers and moralists in spite of all the efforts of the Peace League to suppress it, war will occur, and Universal Peace remain an utopia. The sword will always be of a mighty weight in the balance of the destiny of nations.

But if wars cannot be avoided, could they not be made at least short and decisive? Is not the consideration of the thousands of victims which every war carries with it, a sufficient argument? It would be probably, if every one could be struck with the horrors, with the scenes of suffering and agony, which the military surgeon is daily called to witness.

The statistics of the best organized armies of Europe, where every man is carefully selected by the examining surgeons, and where every thing is provided for the comfort of the soldiers, show that the number of deaths in an army at war is really frightful.

In spite of all the modern implements of war, in spite of the numerous and formidable means of destruction lately adopted, those killed in battle, or who die from wounds, are but a small minority in comparison to those who die from disease.

" In the war with Mexico, the American Army lost but 1549 men in battle and from wounds, whilst 10,986 died from disease in Mexico, besides the hundreds and thousands who returned home to die among their friends from the effects of diseases contracted in camp. " (Chisolm, Manual of Military Surgery.)

We are informed by the same authority that " in the Crimean service, the statistics collected by lord Penmure, Minister of War, show the English loss to have been 22,457, of which number 3,448 were killed in battle, or died from the effects of wounds. Whilst the French loss, as reported to his government by M. Scrive, Inspector General of the French Medical Service in the Crimea, exhibits the frightful loss by death of 63,000 ; whilst the admission into hospital numbered 114,768. This frightful mortality was caused principally by the Asiatic Cholera, which decimated that splendid army.

During the Italian campaign of 1859, the proportion of deaths from wounds as compared with those from diseases was greater than in the Crimean war. It is true that the campaign was short, took place in the best season of the year, in a healthy conntry, where all the necessaries, even luxuries of life were afforded to the troops, and that there were no sieges with all their disastrous consequences. At Solferino, the loss of the Austrians in killed and wounded amounted to 35,000! This frightful loss was chiefly caused by the perfection of the rifled artillery of the French (then used for the first time in battle), which, placed in excellent position, fired 50 shots an hour at a distance of 2,200 metres, with mathematical precision.

When we bear in mind the material of which the armies of this country were composed, when we think that the very large majority of the soldiers were men not trained to the hardships, privations and fatigues of a soldier's life, that they were taken at first promiscuously, without surgical examination, from all classes of society, we readily understand that the mortality among the troops must have been very large. Yet, in spite of all the difficulties under which the armies have been laboring, that mortality, I think, will compare advantageously with that of the armies of Europe.

Dr. Woodward, of the Surgeon General's Bureau at Washington, in his report concerning the mortality of the Federal Army during the first year of the war, ending with June, 1862 says "During this time the general rate of the mortality of our armies was 67,6 per thousand of the average strength of those armies for that year. The rate includes deaths from wounds and injuries, as well as from diseases. The mortality from disease alone was 50,4 per thousand; from wounds and injuries 17,2 per thousand; it thus appears that three of our soldiers die of disease for every one killed in battle. In the Mexican war the mortality rate in our army was 103,8 per thousand, and in the British army during the Crimean War it was 232 per thousand."

During the last two years, from September 1861 to September 1863, not less than 5000 patients were admitted and treated at the Louisiana Hospital of Richmond; this number includes every possible variety of disease and wounds. The general mortality was 11,9 per hundred.

A fact which should be noticed here is the smaller mortality of those hospitals where the kind and devoted hand of women administered to the wants and sufferings of the sick and wounded. After the battles around Richmond, the Louisiana Hospital and one or two others, under the direction of the Sisters of Charity, were publicly cited as having lost much fewer patients than the Government Hospitals, deprived of the zeal and devotion, of such angels of mercy.

Our success at the Louisiana Hospital can also be attributed, in part, to the fact that the patients were treated in a number of small wards, perfectly well ventilated and distributed in large and commodious buildings, one mile from the city, in a most salubrious position, where there was abundance of fresh air and excellent water. All precautions of cleanliness were rigidly enforced; as soon as a case of contagious disease declared itself, it was immediately removed to the "Ward for contagious and eruptive diseases', or to the hospital tents. These I found of invaluable service, a thousand times preferable to the crowded wards of the most palatial buildings, in all cases of an asthœnic character, as well as in the treatment of wounds of the most serious nature, and especially after capital operations; all these cases did infinitely better in tents.

This fact was so well known to the wounded that as soon as their wounds would *begin to look bad* they would themselves ask to be transferred to the tents. These hospital tents are fourteen feet long, fifteen feet wide and eleven feet high in the centre, with a wall four feet and a half high which can be raised for ventilation, and are always protected by a "fly" of appropriate dimension, rendering the tent much more cool and dry; they have a floor elevated several inches from the ground, and which should be covered, when possible, with an oil cloth. Such a tent will accommodate comfortably from 8 to 10 persons. The advantages of this mode of treating wounded men, and those affected with disease of low type, erysipelas, typhus fever, etc., will no doubt astonish many physicians of the old school, who have learned to dread, above all things, the injurious influence of air. To-day, it is proved beyond any doubt, that in the cases alluded to, as well, I might say, as in every case of disease, an abundant supply of pure fresh air is absolutely indispensable; the best directed treatment will often be a complete failure, without the observance of this rule of hygiene. Let your patients—especially your wounded patients—have plenty of air, and guard them above all, from an unrenewed and poisonous atmosphere; the consequences of this would be erysipelas, gangrene, pyœmia and death.

I could mention here several instances of patients having suffered amputations of thigh or arm, resections of the principal joints, who treated in crowded wards, were rapidly sinking under the influence of excessive suppuration, of irritative fever, of pyœmia, who took a sudden change and rapidly recovered, as soon as they were removed to a pure and healthy atmosphere. One of these cases, (a certain Mike Quinn, of a Louisiana Regiment,) with gangrene of the stump, after amputation of the thigh, and sanies of the worst character extending to the groin, where an enormous abcess was formed with numerous fistulas, was removed in a dying condition to a large and well ventilated ward, which was then unoccupied ; there was no change made in the treatment, (brandy, tinct. of iron and bark, stimulants of every kind, tinct. iod. in the fistulas, cauterisation with chlorhydric acid,) etc., which up to the time of his removal, had produced no good result ; that man began to improve as soon as he was placed in a pure atmosphere and after a severe trial of several weeks, recovered perfectly well.

Another important object of consideration in the treatment of wounds, is the dieting of the patients. How many men having suffered operations most skillfully performed by celebrated surgeons, have died from the excessive antiphlogistic diet to which they were submitted, in other words, have been starved to death. In the best organized armies, soldiers suffer from want and exposure ; the fatigues and hardships of active field duty are very great ;—most of the sick soldiers, admitted in the hospitals, after long marches, after several hours, sometimes several days hard fighting, in which they have often been reduced to half, sometimes to one-fourth ration, are completely broken down; they require stimulants, brandy and good food. How much more are these things needed by those wounded who have been prostrated by the loss of blood, by the sufferings of transportation and by excruciating pains! Do not feed such patients, do not restore their strength ready to give way, keep them on tisanes and the mortality among them will be very great. On the contrary give them a good, strong, easily digested, nourrishing diet, let their wants be satisfied, let their appetite be your guide and your success, after capital operations, will be remarkable.

Not many years ago, under the influence of the system of Broussais, bleeding and excessive abstemious diet, amounting to starvation, was the general practice in the treatment of wounds as well as of disease. Since then, modern physicians have gradually abandoned such injurious practice; surgeons have understood the necessity of feeding those who have suffered serious surgical operations; but as it is difficult to eradicate errors and prejudices the proper dieting of patients, of wounded men especially, is far from being generally adopted. A few years ago, while in London, I was much struck with the great difference in the result of operations performed by the French and English surgeons. I then attributed the greater success of the latter, particularly to their generous diet. I recollect having seen in one of the London hospitals a man who had had a leg amputated, to whom was prescribed 2 pints of porter a day, besides other stimulants. The vast opportunity for observation I have lately had leaves no doubt in my mind as to the injurious influence of antiphlogistic treatment (bleeding, etc.) and low diet, in most cases of wounds and especially after surgical operations. — This remark could be applied as well to many cases of disease, especially in this country, where malarial influence predominates, and diseases of low type abound.

During the first part of the war in the autumn of 1861 measles prevailed among the troops. This disease with malarial fevers, diarrhœa and dysentery, filled up the hospitals. Measles, which is generally speaking, a light disease, assumes a more serious character when it assails adults. I observed several cases of a very malignant character, leaving often very serious sequelæ, ophthalmia, diarhœa, bronchitis, persistent otorrhœa, which could be cured only with great difficulty. — These sequelæ kept a large number of young recruits in the hospitals during the whole winter months. As it is always the case with an army, in the beginning of a campaign, the number of the sick and the dead was far greater during the first months than later, when the recruits had become accustomed to the hardships of camp life. — To become a soldier, it requires a regular training, the ordeal of which is not passed successfully by all. In this country where armies had to be improvised, that want of routine was sorely felt. Not accustomed to the work, privations, hardships and fatigues to which they were, without any transition, compelled to submit, new soldiers were rapidly seized with disease, and a severe attack generally proved fatal.

I have but little to say in relation to the diseases which prevailed during the first period of the war. Quinine in moderate doses, in cases of malarial fevers, opium, calomel and ipecac and light astringents in diarrhæa and dysentery, generally proved very successful. — Quinine in small doses, 2 or 3 gr. combined with a very small quantity of opium, 1/6 grain, given every morning, for 2 or 3 weeks as prophylactic, prevented, almost in every case, the return of the fever after it had been once checked. I have seen persons who had been for months and months the victims of intermittent fever, returning under the least exposure, remain entirely safe, and protected from new attacks, under the influence of this treatment, although they continued to reside in parts of the country where malaria prevailed.

As to the treatment of measles, besides light diaphoretics and other usual treatment, I would strongly recommend in every case the use of Liq. acet. ammoniæ (spiritus mindereri) which given in doses of 40 or 50 drops, 3 times a day, in a cup of warm tea, seems to possess a particular eliminating action. — Even in the sequelæ of Rubeola, I have found it very useful. — I am inclined to consider it as possessing specific properties in Rubeola. It was the principal medicinal agent used by my father, several years ago, in the cure of a case of deafness, following a very severe attack of measles. The patient was a son of Mr Martin Dural of this city, and success was complete.

During the months of December 1861 and January 1862, typhoid fever and pneumonia prevailed almost epidemically in the hospitals of Richmond. At that time these two diseases, the latter especially, killed more soldiers than any other. — Men affected with acute pneumonia in its full development, were sent from the field, over rough roads, in the most inclement months of the year, from a long distance, to the Richmond hospitals where they very often arrived in a hopeless condition.

In typhoid fever, experience soon proved us that all depressing agents were to be carefully avoided, and that the asthænic character of the disease was to be remembered.—Saline purgatives (Delarroques method) followed by stimulants, and meeting besides the most alarming symptoms as they occured, proved the most efficacious treatment.—In cases where there was much tympanitis, dryness, and fuliginous condition of the tongue and fauces, gurgle and pain in right fossa iliaca, and moderate diarrhæa, the oleum terebenthinœ had an excellent effect; when there was any marked remission in the symptoms, quinine was given with advantage. Frequent sponging of the body with water and vinegar was of great comfort. During the convalescence of typhoid fever, as well as of most diseases of long duration, the tinct muriat. ferri was found to be the best tonic, improving rapidly the condition of the blood.

In pneumonia, dry or scarified cupping according to the general condition of the patient, which very often prohibited absolutely blood letting, followed by very large blisters on the chest, expectorants combined with chlorhydrate of ammonia, 5 grains every 3 hours and often with carb. ammonia, proved to be the best treatment. In almost every case, the patient was put on strong beef tea, milk punch, etc. The tartar emetic in large doses and other preparations of antimony, so useful in civil practice, were not admissible, extreme prostration immediately following in all the cases in which they were used. But emetic given simply to promote vomiting, or ipecac, had an excellent effect when administered in the first period of the disease. Our practice confirms the greater gravity of inflammation of the left lung, when compared to that of the right. Bleeding was generally found more injurious than useful ; I have already mentioned the prostrated condition of the men who usually reached the hospital after several days sickness. In almost every case of disease that came under my observation, debility very soon made its appearance, and stimulants had to be given very freely ; brandy which I had seldom used in civil practice, proved a most valuable medicine. It is especially in cases of pneumonia observed in military hospitals, that a physician can see how different must be the treatment of the same disease, according to the condition of the patient, the different locality, mode of life, etc., things that have been known for a long time, and which experience confirms every day.

I have but little to say in relation to the other medical diseases which reigned in the hospitals of Richmond during the spring and summer of 1862. Diarrhœa, dysentery (generally of a mild form) and gastric disturbance continued to be the prevailing diseases. They were generally the result of suppression of perspiration and of intemperance in eating and drinking. — Unripe fruits and vegetables, indigestible food of every kind, poisonous whiskey will always be the great temptation of soldiers. — We had many cases of camp fever, so called, because it generally accompanies armies ; it is considered by many surgeons as typhus fever. — I found it very different from the real typhus I had observed in Italy. This is a much more serious disease, and always produces great mortality among the troops — it is always the result of animal emanations. Camp fever which I observed in Virginia was rather a form of typhoid fever, of less duration; abdominal symptoms predominated instead of the cerebral which are predominating in typhus fever; the treatment was generally successful and consisted especially in the use of opium and stimulating tonics.

In the month of April 1862, after several months training and military preparations on both sides, began in Virginia a series of bloody battles and serious engagements which has continued with but very little remission, up to the present day. At that time, the hospitals began to be crowded with wounded of all sorts, and they have since formed the principal portion of the inmates of the hospitals.

It is curious to notice after each great battle, how suddenly all other cases of disease, disappear to make room for the wounded. These alone attract attention, excite interest and sympathy, the others sink in insignificance; nobody seems to care any more for the poor fellow who lies—afflicted with diarrhœa or fever—close to a soldier who has lost either an arm or leg on the battle field, and who with a flash in his eyes, relates with enthusiasm the different phases of the battle. Strange human nature! These two men have both suffered for the same cause, both will perhaps give it their life, and yet how differently they are looked upon. The wounded man is regarded as a hero, whilst the other is scarcely noticed. The sympathy excited by a bleeding limb, by something which makes an impression on our mind through our senses will always be stronger than that which is excited by a disease we do do not see and which we know nothing about.

Before speaking of the several rare and interesting cases of wounds which I had the opportunity of noticing, and the different operations they required, I will say a few words of a disease of the most serious character, which carried off large numbers of soldiers, during the autumn and winter of 1862. I allude to small pox which was said to have been imported in the Southern Army, by prisoners of war, returning from the North where it reigned considerably. Its first origin was attributed to the fact of these prisoners having slept one night, on their way home, in a house (I cannot remember the name of the locality) which had been used shortly before as a small pox hospital by the Northern troops.— The first cases of this loathsome disease were observed, I think, in the month of September and spreaded gradually until it assailed a very large number of soldiers. A large small pox Hospital was established in Richmond, at Howard's Grove, at a considerable distance from the City, in an elevated and salubrious position, and all the other hospitals received orders to have all their varioloid and variola cases removed immediately to this Howard's Grove Hospital. Vaccinations and revaccinations were practiced in the whole army, as soon as the first cases of small pox made their appearance. I do not know what has been the mortality caused by this frightful disease in the hospitals of Richmond, and in the army in general; I have however reasons to believe that it has not been as great, as it is generally under similar circumstances. At the Louisiana Hospital, we had 13 cases, 8 of true variola, and 5 of varioloid. They were all treated in a separate building removed at a considerable distance from the main buildings, and no communication was allowed between them.

The utmost cleanliness was observed, chlorine fumigations were made daily and all other hygienic principles strictly enforced. But above all, we insisted upon thorough *ventilation* of the wards, for we are of opinion with a large number of modern surgeons, that *air* is the *only* true desinfecting agent, and that, without it, all the others are of no value. Out of 13 cases of small pox, we lost 4, one of whom (F. Taylor, of the 9th La. Regt.) had organic disease of the heart, and another (Dan. Joyne, of the 1st La.,) had suffered two amputations of thigh ; he was progressing very favorably after the second operation, performed at the hospital (the first was performed on the battle field ; the lesions of the bone extending several inches above the line of section, it was necessary to re-amputate) when he was suddenly taken with variola which in a few days carried him to his grave. Private J. K. Stewart, of Comp. C. 2d La. Regt., was just recovering from his numerous wounds, compound fracture of right fore arm and left fibula, besides three flesh wounds, when he was taken sick with small pox which fortunately, was not very severe. In spite of his debilitated condition he recovered perfectly well.

Our treatment consisted principally in saline purgatives, cooling drinks, and enemata in the view of abating the force of the eruptive fever and keeping down the number of pustules when these were confluent; in cases in which the eruption seemed deficient, the liq. acet. ammmon. readily promoted it. Opiates given once or twice a day had an excellent effect in moderating the restlessness, tremors and delirium which generally occured.

During the period of suppuration, the strength of the patient was supported by a nourishing diet, by wines and cordials, and liquor. sodæ. chlorinatæ. administered internally in view of its antisceptic properties. The eyes were carefully washed with water and vinegar, — and the pustules of the eye lids touched with the lunar caustic to prevent dangerous ophthalmia. — As to the prevention of the pitting or seaming of the face, which was not so important in our class of patients, mercurial ointment smeared from time to time, was the only thing used.

Before coming to that part of our observations which refers to gun shot wounds and to the operations they required, I will speak *en passant* of a few surgical cases of daily occurence in civil practice.

Among many others, I could mention a case of urinary infiltration, from stricture, extending to the upper internal part of thighs, to the perineum, scrotum and abdominal parietes up to the umbilicus, and complicated with an enormous inguinal hernia of years standing. This case occured in an old man (Amy Leroy, of the 10th La. Regiment), and was successfully treated by numerous deep incisions, (12), one opening the whole length of the scrotum, half of which mortified, by injections of pure tinct. iod. and Labarraque solution, and introduction of catheter in the bladder; tinct. chloridi ferri iu large doses internally 20 drops every two hours] tonics and stimulants,—This old man, after being on the verge of death [extreme prostration, diarrhæ a, hectic fever] completely recovered.

One case of radical cure of Inguinal Hernia by Weirtzer's method (Robert Magee. 6th La.); the operation failed in two other cases, of many years standing and in which the rings of the canal were very much dilated.

One case of complicated fracture of skull [D. C. Clough 5th La Co I] from blows and injuries received in a street fight,—A large piece of the left parietalis bone was detached and extracted— most violent cerebritis took place. The patient was twice saved from imminent death by the application of a large blister covering the whole scalp.

Finally, several cases of varix cured by the injection in the veins of per chloride of iron, a large number of ablations of hemorrhoidal tumors by the "Ecraseur", etc.

About one half of our operations were *secondary*: that is, were performed after suppuration was established. Now every surgeon knows that an operation performed in the first 24 hours that follow the injury, before febrile reaction sets in (primary), is much more apt to succeed than an operation performed at any other period.

There seems to be but one exception to this rule; resection at the hip joint is more successful when secondary than when primary, although the success in neither case, is far from being very satisfactory. In the Histoire Medico Chirurgicale de la Guerre de Crimée par le docteur Adolphe Armand, we find that out of 36 primary resections at the hip joint after gun shot wounds, but one was cured, and 35 died; out of 12 secondary resections at the same joint, 3 were saved and 9 died. It is also generally admitted that amputations rendered necessary by traumatic lesions are more dangerous than those we perform for chronic organic lesions; in other word, that an operation performed for disease succeeds better than one performed for injury. Out of 24 amputations for organic alterations, in young subjects from five to fifteen, 8 deaths, 16 cures; for traumatic lesions, out of 4 amputations, 4 deaths. (Malgaigne, archives générales de médecine, avril 1842.)

Among the successful amputations of thigh performed at the Louisiana Hospital of Richmond is one in the upper third, (secondary) which so seldom proves satisfactory; here is the observation:

L. Dwyer, private, 14th La. Regt. Comp. F. entered the hospital July 1st 1862. Wounded at Gaines Mill, on the 27th June, at the union of the upper and middle third of right thigh. When he entered the hospital, his leg was in a fracture box, he suffered but very little, and we had no idea of the gravity of the case until several days after, when the fever having subsided, and the suppurative process being well established, we probed the wound with the finger, which revealed terrible lesions. There was but one opening in the anterior upper part of the thigh; it was small, regular, linear, and resembled more an incised wound than a gun shot wound; it led directly to the bone which was crushed; numerous spiculœ of all sizes and dimensious were distinctly felt; a very sharp pointed fragment extended downwards beyond the reach of the finger, a buck shot was extracted with the forceps from the wound. The projectile(what was it)? was probably lodged in the bone. A consultation was held with Dr. W. C. Nichols, of this city, and we both came to the conclusion, that the lesion was such as to necessitate the immediate amputation. The patient was yonng, strong and vigorous. The circular amputation was immediately performed (July 8th) the incision of the integuments included the bullet hole so little tissue was there left above to cover the bone. The fracture was found not to extend, very fortunately, above the opening of the projectile, but several large fragments extended downwards to 4 inches above the knee joint; the bone was completely crushed; two heavy pieces of lead, flattened and irregular, and three buck shots were found lodged among the fragments. — This man recovered perfectly well, after a long and profuse suppuration during which his strength was sustained by tonics and stimulants; he was keeping a fruit store in Richmond when I left.

This may be considered as an exceptional case; in the great majority of cases, amputations in the upper third of thigh are fatal. In the Crimea all those that were amputated in the vicinity of the trochanter died. Baudens blames amputation in the superior third of thigh. His experience proves that in compound fracture of upper portion of thigh, more patients are saved, when attempts are made to save the limb, than after amputation. He succeeded by the use of the fracture box and inclined plane in saving a patient who had a compound fracture on a level with the trochanter, although he had extracted two inches of the shaft of the femur. In a similar case, I also extracted 2 inches of bone immediately below the trochanter, but was not so fortunate; the patient died 3 days after.

If there is any doubt as to the propriety of amputating in the upper portion of thigh in compound comminutive fracture, there can be none when the lesion exists in the inferior portion. Every surgeon knows that the dangers of operations diminish as they are performed at a greater distance from the trunk. If attempts are made to save the limb, the chances of death will be almost as great as in compound fracture of the superior portion (the majority will die after excessive sufferings), especially in military hospitals where exist so many unfavorable circumstances, while by amputation many will be saved.

I will remark here that amputations in general seem to be less successful in our days than formerly. This is probably due to the difference in the projectiles now used, compared to those of former years. In fact the conical ball (which causes more deaths and wounds than other apparently more frightful projectiles of war) produces much more crushing and comminution, much more splitting of the bones, extending often to the joints, than the round ball, the nervous shock is consequently greater, and that may have some influence in the results of amputation. I have seen a man, who had received a gun shot wound (Minié) which had penetrated and shattered the knee joint, die less than two hours after the injury, from the shock — there was no hemorrhage; the patient remained pale, cold and faint, with weak, irregular, tremulous pulse, and want of conciousness, until he died.

After the terrible naval engagement which took place June 1st 1794, Dr. Fercoc, surgeon major of the vessel le *Jemmape*, wrote to Larrey, that out of 66 primary amputations, 2 alone died from tetanus: one of these had had his two arms amputated. — after the engagement of Neuberg, Percy performed 92 amputations, 86 recovered; Larrey cured 12 out of 14. — After the battle of New Orleans in 1815, out of 45 primary amputations, 38 recovered (Guthrie).

It was after an amputation of thigh that I observed the only case of tetanus that occured in the hospital. This formidable complication declared itself in a young, healthy subject, 14 days after the operation, apparently without any cause, when every thing was progressing favorably.

Our mortality after amputation of the superior extremities was 1/8; after amputation of inferior extremities 1/5. These amputations were necessitated by comminutive fracture, especially in the lower extremities, by wounds implicating large joints, by mortification, finally, when after an attempt at saving a fractured limb or a perforated joint, life was threatened by continued irritation and excessive suppuration. I always preferred the circular method to any other, on account of its leaving less sof parts to suppurate to slough, thereby diminishing the dangers of the operation, and of its mor rapid cicatrization.

In all our operations, we invariably used chloroform, and although its full effect was obtained, and that period of *tolerance*, as Dr CHASSAIGNAC of Paris, calls it, reached in every case, we never met with the least accident or even inconvenience. I consider it of *utmost importance* that an operation should never be *begun* while the patient is still in the period of *excitement*, as I have frequently seen it done. During this period. the nervous power of the patient is *considerably* increased, several strong men are required to hold him, his muscles are all in spasmodic contraction and sensibility is far from being abolished.

The Surgeon who refuses his patient the full benefit of

this most wonderful agent, of this blessing of God, is barbarous, ignorant and not worthy of his age. — Do not operate until your patient is fully under the influence of chloroform, untill the period of anæsthesia, of complete insensibility is reached. That period can be protracted more or less, for an indefinite time, by renewing at intervals the inhalation of chloroform.

During the Italian campaign, I saw cases of traumatic tetanus, in which the patient was kept under its influence for ten and twelve hours. In England, women are daily delivered under the influence of chloroform. By administering it with proper precautions (the patient being placed *horizontally*, the head not higher than the body, the first inhalations being well diluted with air, etc.), by being guided *exclusively* by the effects of this powerful agent in each individual case, the dose required to produce anæsthesia varying infinitely, you will have no cause to fear any accident. In the Crimea, chloroform was administered in more than 60,000 cases and never caused a single accident, and still we find, as Chisolm so verily remarks, some of the old school, who are in authority, sneer at its pretensions and magnify its dangers.

Eight resections at the shoulder joint, two at the elbow, one at the wrist, and one in the continuity of the humerus were performed and treated at the Louisiana Hospital.

They all succeeded remarkably well, with the exception of one at the shoulder joint, in which case the desarticulation ought to have been performed at first, instead of the resection, as will be seen by the observation at the end; the patient recovered with the loss of his arm. In all the other cases the patients regained a very useful limb.

Resections at the shoulder-joint gave excellent results; the patients, besides running much less danger than in the desarticulation, recovered with limbs possessing all the motions with the exception of the deltoid, which muscle remained more or less paralized, on account of the inevitable division of some of its nerves.

All cases of gun shot wounds interesting large joints that came under my observation required either resection or amputation; — I at first attempted to save life without operation, by cupping, leeching, bold incisions in the joint to give exit to the pus, cold irrigation, etc. but with no good result. Apparently trifling injuries were followed by excessive inflammation with destruction of the whole joint. Resection is more applicable to the superior than to the inferior extremities; amputations of the latter will always be more frequent. In the arm, sensibility and mobility are much more essential than solidity which is absolutely required in the inferior extremities to sustain and carry forward the body; considerable extent of the bones of the upper extremity can be removed without rendering the limb useless; whatever may be the shortening after resection, if the hand is saved *that* alone is of an *immense* advantage, while the least shortening of the leg has very great inconveniences.

Resection ought to be performed in preference to amputation in every case of compound fracture (gun shot) of arm, where the nerves and arteries are not injured nor the soft parts extensively lacerated. When the bone is not extensively crushed, an attempt ought to be made to save the limb, without operation. Paste board and gutta percha splints, moulding themselves perfectly to the shape of the limb are very useful in this case. Spiculœ should be immediately extracted and the wounds left open to give free exit to the pus. — By following this course, I succeeded in several instances to save the limb without any deformity.— Among others, I will only mention here Lieut. Johnson of the 5th La. Regt., who recovered from severe compound fracture of upper portion of humerus, with perfect use of limb, and without any deformity.

In injury of the hip joint, resection should also be preferred to desarticulation which proves speedily fatal in the immense majority of cases. In the Crimea not a single coxo femoral desarticulation proved successful while the result was a little more satisfactory in cases of resection. —They saved 1 in 6, and would have saved more, had the general conditions of the troops been better. (Chisolm.)

The dangers of resection compared to those of amputation are much less. — In the Schleswig-Holstein army, out of 54 amputations of the arm 19 died, whilst, out of 40 resections under similar circumstances only 6 died.

The reader will find hereafter the detailed observation of a case of resection at the elbow joint (Capt. H. Myatt's) followed with extraordinary success.

The principal rules for all resections are that the incisions made to reach the injured bones should be performed on that side of the limb where there are no important blood vessels and nerves, that they should be sufficiently long to expose and dissect easily the heads of the bones. It is recommended besides that as much periosteum, and as little synovial membrane as possible should be retained, the first is necessary to the formation of new bone, the second is apt to inflame. No reunion by first intention is to be expected; suppuration will generally be profuse and long continued; guard against *debility;* give your patient good nourishment and stimulants.— Use cold water dressing and apply no bandage, no splint of any sort to the limb until healthy granulations fill up the cavity caused by the extraction of the bones, it will then be time to apply the tumefaction bandage for removing the œdema of the limb, and the necessary lspints (paste board or gutta percha,) and also to guard against anchylosis, by passive motions in the pseudo-joint. As soon as fever has subsided, and suppuration is well established, the patient should be permitted to leave his bed.

Several cases of desarticulation at the shoulder joint (flap and ovalar method) performed on the battle field, were treated at the hospital, and not a single one died. A tibio-tarseal desarticulation (D. LEBLANC, of the Donaldsonville Artillery) and a desarticulation of Chopart (E. TURCK, Comp. C. 7th La. Regt.) had also excellent results.

At this hospital I always prescribed that the dressing of wounds should be extremely simple discarding as much as possible lint, charpie and bandages which used to be considered indispensable. I at first did so from necessity, lint and linen were scarce articles,— but I soon found that a simple compresse wet in cold water and often renewed was more advantageous than elegant bandages which kept the parts warm and irritated. — Wounds cicatrize much better and sooner by the water dressing. Cold irrigation was used with utmost advantage in all cases where violent inflammation threatened or existed. — After operations, the wound was united by means of the suture, and no adhesive plaster used. I cannot say that I ever witnessed a case of union by first intention after a capital operation, but frequently saw wounds heal with but very little suppuration. In almost every case, the flabby condition of the wounds required some stimulant and astringent application; solution of nitrate of silver more or less concentrated, and tincture iodine were generally used with benefit in promoting healthy granulation. In cases where there was much fœtor, the liquor sodæ chlorinatœ (Labarraque's solution) was invariably used.

A small number of penetrating wounds of the chest were treated at the hospital, the majority of those wounds causing immediate death and not bearing transportation from the field. I however had the opportunity of seeing several cases of gun shot wounds *of the lung* in which the patient was saved.

M. Kennedy, 19 years old, [Comp. D. 1st La. Regiment] wounded near Richmond on the 21st June 1862.—The ball [Minié] entered the chest on the left side, between the 9th and 10th rib in front, and was extracted two weeks after, in the back, 1 1|2 inch from the spine, opposite the 8th rib.—There was hemorrhage from the mouth, from the wounds, escape of air, etc.—This patient recovered with hernia of the lung, protruding under the skin, between the 9th and 10th rib in front, of the size of a pigeon's egg.—His general condition was good.

In cases of penetrating wounds of the chest venœsection finds its most useful application; it often checks internal hemorrhage, which otherwise would have been speedily fatal, diminishes dyspnœa and infllammation. Opium should be given freely and frequently, it quiets the cough, diminishes respiration, allays pain, and by its antiphlogistic properties operates directly against inflammation ; digitalis and veratrum viride should also be given to controle the action of the heart. Ice should be used freely internally and externally. The patient should lie on the wounded side.

If profuse hemorrhage is caused by the lesion of an artery which can be reached such as the intercostal, or the internal mamary (this very seldom occurs) the wound should be enlarged and the bleeding vessel ligated. McLeod states that during the crimean war, he neither saw nor heard of an instance of injury to the intercostal artery.

When the hemorrhage does not proceed from the lesion of these arteries, the wound should be accurately closed. The blood coagulating in the cavity of the chest will compress the bleeding vessels, and hemorrhage will generally cease. Besides, the closure of the wound will exclude the introduction of air which would cause the decomposition of extravasated fluids, and will to a cerain degree, prevent emphysema.

It is only in cases of imminent suffocation, or when the presence of suppuration (empyema) threatens to destroy life, that the wound should be dilated or the thorax opened to give free exit to the pent up fluids.

The presence of foreign bodies (which is more than probable in shot wounds of the chest, when there is but one orifice and the clothing has been perforated) will add greatly to the dangers of such wounds; sharp spiculæ from fractured ribs are the most dangerous. The search made for them should however not be too protracted, and no probe used except the finger.

When no' easily detected, the wound should be closed with diachylon and the general treatment insisted upon. Their presence is not *absolutely* incompatible with life, not even with health. Several examples are recorded in surgical books, of men having lived for number of years with enkysted balls or other foreign bodies remaining in the lung.

The most extraordinary case of penetrating wound is the following :

GUN SHOT WOUND,

PENETRATING RIGHT LUNG AND LIVER;—RECOVERY.

JULIEN ARNAUD, 21 years old, of the 15th La. Regt. Comp. K. was admitted at the Louisiana Hospital of Richmond, May 13th 1863; wounded at Chancellorsville May 3d, by a Minié ball entering the right hypochondriac region in front, at the point of union of the cartilages of the 8th and 9th rib, and coming out behind opposite the 1lth rib which it fractured, at 4 inches from the spine. Shortly after the injury, considerable hemorrhage from the mouth as well as from the wounds, ceasing spontaneously during the night; for 3 or 4 days he continued to to spit blood.

On admittance (May 13th) the patient was very much troubled by hiccup and vomiting which had lasted for 5 days; complete prostration; constant and hacking cough, expectoration, after much effort, of pure bile; bile comes out also in quantity from the 2 openings; stools liquid and whitish, but regular; the patient had vomited all the food he had taken for the last 4 days.

Diagnosis: Gun shot wound penetrating the liver and base of right lung.

Ice was prescribed in small pieces, constantly kept in the mouth and swallowed — the patient took it with avidity. In the afternoon vomiting ceased and iced weak brandy toddy was prescribed. This was the only nourishment for two days. Pulse weak and frequent; no pains except when coughing — sleep regular — great dullness at the base of the lung; auscultation impossible on account of the incessant cough. The wounds were dressed with dry charpie applied in thick layers and always found saturated with bile, at each dressing, 3 and 4 times a day.

May 16th. Less bile in the secretions which are getting more purulent; no vomiting; prostration much less; cough still frequent and sputa assuming a mucous character. — At the evening dressing a small spicula is extracted in the posterior wound. Ice and punch are continued, with the addition of beef-tea, milk and soup.

May 21st. Patient complains of pains along the false ribs; some diarrhæa; whitish stools: 1 grain of opium every 4 hours and starch injections.

May 21st. Diarrhæa almost ceased; secretion by the anterior wound very much diminished; while the wounds are being dressed, a bubble of air comes out with *noise* from the posterior wound; expectoration which does not contain any more bile, and cough, are less — the patient sleeps well at night, and takes more nourishment and stimulants. The passages still liquid have regained their natural colour.

The amelioration is kept up regularly to the 10th June. At that time fever supervenes, the cough increases, the sputa become rusty, and aulscultation reveals partial pneumonia of the inferior part of right lung. For several days the patient takes with benefit small doses of opium and calomel. On disappearance of acute pulmonary symptoms, chlorhydrate of ammonia is prescribed (20 gr. in 4 doses a day) and also the Muriat. Tinct, Iron (15 drops 3 times a day. The sal ammoniac is continued for 8 days, and the tincture of iron for seral weeks. — The patient improves. On the 28th he walks about the yard; his appetite is good and he is gaining his stregth.

In the first part of July, the wounds are completely closed; no more cough, all the functions are natural. — The right inferior part of the thorax is very convex; the 9th rib is separated from its cartilaginous attach with the 8th, and the anterior margin of the 10th rib can be easily felt under the abdominal parietes, about 2 1/2 inches above the superior edge of the iliac bone (cresta iliaca). Air penetrates the right lung in its two superior thirds. Two months after, I had the opportunity of seeing Julien Arnaud; he was in excellent health.

In general hospital No. 1, in charge of Dr. Gibson, (Richmond) I observed a case of gun shot wound of lung with emphysema extending to three-fourths of the whole body !

In one instance, I observed a partial paralysis of the inferior extremities, after a gun shot wound of thorax [not penetrating]. The ball [Minié] had entered near the external margin of the right scapula and deeply lodged itself near the vertebral column, so at least it was supposed, for the ball was not to be found. The external wound healed without any trouble, but the patient (General Joseph Johnston wounded at the battle of Seven Pines, near Richmond,) remained for a long time unable to ride or walk any distance, even with the help of a stick. — Falling from his horse, in receiving that wound, the general had besidos broken one of his inferior right ribs. — There was no pain; the general health was good, but the patient complained of extreme weakness in his legs, with sensibility somewhat diminished, and motions greatly impaired. — What was the cause of this semi-paralysis which existed for at least two months ? It would have beeu necessary to know the exact seat of the ball, and that could not be ascertained; some time before I saw the patient, an incision had been made to find out the ball, which still remained.—The most careful examination could no where discover it. I prescribed cold shower baths on the spine, and strychnia internally [1-12 grain twice a day] and externally.

This treatment — " *un peu aveugle* " — had the best results. — I had attended the General at Amélia Springs.— Three or four weeks after, he walked one morning from Richmond to the hospital and back [over two miles.]— He had completely recovered the use of his legs, could ride very well, and was preparing to take the field.

We observed but few wounds of the abdomen, these wounds being generally too serious to bear transportation. It was in a wound of this kiud in which the ball had entered two inches below the umbilicus and had ranged downwards in the thickness of the parietes towards the left horizontal ramus of the pubis, there remaining, that I experienced for the first time the instrument imagined by Professor Nélaton, of Paris, at the time he was called to La Spezia, to visit Garibaldi and decide whether the ball was remaining in the Dictator's foot or not. The object of the instrument is to detect, in doubtful cases, whether a ball is remaining or not in a wound. The instrument I used, was Luer's modification of Nélaton's and had just been brought from Paris, by my friend Dr. Estorge of Opelousas.—It consists of a hollow canula of the size of an ordinary grooved conductor, through which moves a probe (une tige) terminated at its end in two small branches shaped like a spoon, with cutting edges capable of cutting or scraping a small particle of lead, when pressing directly against the ball. When the instrument is withdrawn from the *trajet* of the wound, and a small parcel of lead is found in the spoons, there is no doubt as to the presence of the projectile; but this may remain in the wound and not be detected by the exploring instrument, for instance, if the projectile be of some other metal than lead, if it be surrounded with coagula, with a piece of cloth or other foreign substance, etc. The instrument is, I think, more ingenious than really useful. The surgeon's finger will always be the best and surest guide, the only one upon which he can rely; without it, it is impossible in most cases, to have a correct idea of the amount of injury.

This examination of a wound should always be made

before reaction sets in and as soon as possible after the injury or when suppuration is well established.

Penetrating wounds of abdomen are as dangerous as those of the chest. They should never be probed, except to ascertrin whether the wound is penetrating or not, this circumstance making all the difference in the gravity of the case; and foreign bodies that have penetratred beyond the abdominal parietes should not be searched for. Chisolm very wisely remarks that in all perforating wounds of the abdomen, as we cannot tell, in the absence of symptoms, whether the intestines have been injured or not, there are two fundamental rules of treatment never to be forgotten, aud which are required in every instance :

1 °. Give opium freely and frequently, with a double object, viz: of controlling the peristaltic action, which alone can prevent extravasation of the contents into the peritoneal cavity; and for its antiphlogistic effect, to equalize the circulation, allay pain, suspend nervous irritability, and prevent inflammation.

2 °. Avoid the use of purgatives.

For three or four days at least after the occurence of injury, in which the intestines are known, or are *supposed* to be wounded, absolute rest, the most abstemious diet, and the liberal use of opium (1 grain of gum opium every 4 hours) in connection with cold water or iced dressing, will compose the entire treatment.

Should the intestines be perforated, which is proved

by the escape of fœcal matter) they should be carefully closed with suture ; should they be extensively injured, they should be left in the external opening — hoping that adhesions will take place, and an artificial anus will form; the injured portion of the intestine has sometimes been excised, the intestine sewed and reintroduced in the cavity of the abdomen, the patient recovering. Dr GASTON of Columbia, S. C. had under his charge a lunatic who attempted suicide by opening his abdomen, drawing out his bowels, and cutting off two feet of intestine. The two ends of the intestines were brought together, secured by carefully arranged sutures, aud returned within the abdomen. The patient made a perfect recovery (Chisolm.)

In case of hemorrhage from the division of the epigastric or mesenteric the wound should be dilated, and the arteries ligated.

The treatment of gun shot wounds of the abdominal viscera or blood vessels is on the whole entirely unsatisfactory, and the large majority are fatal.

Among the observations given at the end will be found an interesting case of gun shot wound of the bladder.

I had also the opportunity of treating several cases of gun shot wounds of the genitals with considerable infiltration, ecchymosis, darkish hue and enormous swelling ; these lesions, so serious, in appearance, generally healed very quickly. In one case, the urethra was perforated by a Minié ball which penetrated the scrotum without injuring the spermatic chord or testicle, and lodged itself in the perineum, one inch from the anus — the ball was extracted, a catheter intoduced into the bladder, the wounds healed without leaving a fistula. In an other case, in which the loss of substance of the urethra was considerable, there remained a fistulous opening which au autoplastic operation afterwards cured perfectly. I never observed any hemorrhage from these wounds.

In a third case, the scrotum was transfixed by a ball which lodged itself in the inner part of the thigh ; the spermatic chord was cut, and the testicle suffered complete atrophy; its size was reduced to that of a bean. The testicle was uninjured in all the cases I saw.

I shall now say a few words of gun shot wounds of the head. These are always serious, hewever trivial they may appear. *Nullum vulnus capitis læve* is an aphorism which must be borne in mind. The slightest injury sometimes gives rise to violent inflammation of the brain. In wounds of the scalp without injury to the bone as well as in compound fracture of skull (shot wound) with or without depression, the surgeon will insist upon the antiphlogistic treatment rest, quiet, etc. I have seen repeatedly the free use of the lancet relieve threatening symptoms of compression from extravasation of blood.

In concussion of the brain, in which there is momentary suspension of the functions of this organ, unless the pulse be feeble and intermittent, or the insensibility and the unconciousness too protracted, leave the case to nature, be satisfied with dashing a little cold water on the face, and avoid giving stimuli as they would increase the effusion of blood in case the brain be lacerated. Like syncope, concussion will sometimes save life ; if blood vessels have been torn, condition which is at first ignored, *during concussion*, the blood may have coagulated, and hemorrhage, always so serious, may by that means be avoided.

Bleeding shall never be used in ***concussion***, it would be sure to hasten death.

This conditicn may be accompanied with more or less extensive lesions of the cerebral mass, congestion, extravasion, laceration, etc. In some instances, although the concussion has been strong enough to produce instantaneous death, no lesions of any kind have been found in the brain. It is impossibls at first to diagnose the pathological condition of the brain ; after the patient has recovered from the shock, we should watch carefully his condition, place him in a cool room, use cold water on his head, avoid all stimulants and wait for the symptoms. If the lesion has not been such as to produce laceration and extravasation in the substance of the brain, the patient will gradually recover; should symptoms of compression declare themselves, the surgeon should insist upon a general and local antiphlogistic treatment; bleeding, cupping, bladder filled with ice or cold irrigation on the head, purgatives, etc.

Compression is to be feared for several days and even weeks after the injury, it may be caused either by extravasated blood,, by portion of the skull, or some foreign body making pressure upon the cerebral mass. Its symptoms are coma, stupor, paralysis general or local, according to the seat and extent of the part which is compressed, stertorous and blowing breathing, — "*le malade fume la pipe*"—slow and full pulse, pupils dilated and insensible to light.—Unless the causes of compression be removed, this state generally very soon terminates fatally.

Trephine was formerly considered the proper treatment in similar cases. —It was performed at the seat of injury, for there the cause of compression (either bone, foreign body or extravasated blood) was expected to be found. But it often occurred that the operation was useless; the lesions existed in some other part of the skull, a blood vessel had been torn in an opposite point to that of injury, or portion of the skull, or the ball had been driven into the cerebral substance too far from the external wound to be reached. It is unecessary to remark that unless the foreign body is superficial, and easily detected, it would be madness to probe the brain. Modern military surgeons are generally greatly opposed to trephining, except in cases of compound fracture, with depressed fragments, existing in connection with symptoms of compression; even in those cases the propriety of trephining is doubted by many of vast experience —who think that the loose fragments of bone should be simply extracted and antiphlogistic treatment insisted upon. Chisolm is of opinion that " the operation of trephining is always very serious *per se*, and is sufficient of itself to cause cerebral or meningeal inflammation which will nearly always terminate fatally.

The operation is often more serious than the condition for which it is used, and although the patient might recover from either, he succumbs under the combination. Experience and autopsies have shown us many cases of extensive intra cranial hemorrhages, which have been unaccompanied by symptoms denoting such an accident, and the traces of such have been found when the patient recovering from his head injury, had fallen a victim to some totally foreign disease. Had such a condition been suspected, and the surgeon used his instruments, an autopsy at a much earlier day would have revealed the condition."

Stromyer, one of the best authorities on gun shot wouuds of the head, which he has particularly studied, says in a work recently published "*that in military surgery trephining is never needed.*" When the case is so serious as to require the trephine in gun shot wounds, the patient will die in spite of it. Lœffler, a distinguished surgeon in the Prussian service, McLeod, who had great experience in the Crimea, Hewett and many other modern surgeons are equally opposed to trephining.

The entire records of the science may be searched in vain, to find a duplicate series of successful cases to that reported by Stromyer. Of forty one cases of fracture with depression from gun shot wounds, in many of which it was probable that the brain and membranes were injured, only seven died. All the rest recovered. In only *one* case was there any operative interference, *although signs of sécondary compression appeared in several.* The anti-phlogistic treatment, carefully carried out, was alone adhered to. (Chisolm). To have a better view of the remarkable success of Stromyer, it must be recollected that of ninety one cases of penetrating and perforating gun shot wounds of the head which were admitted into hospital in the Crimea, all, without exception, proved fatal.

For my part, in the treatment of gun shot wounds of head which came under my observations, I strictly carried out the views of Stromyer and other modern surgeons, and out of 12 cases of compound fracture of skull, the ball remaining in one instance partly embedded in the surface of the brain, I was fortunate enough to save nine patients. I will give hereafter an observation of gun shot wound of the head, with loss of both eyes, and another of compound fracture of os frontalis from gun-shot, followed by meningitis and erysipelas ;—both cases recovered.

It has been often questioned whether the conical ball followed the contour of bones without causing any fracture, as does so frequently the round ball. Although I have seen this but seldom, yet cases have occurred to me in which the conical ball described exactly the contour of the skull without causing fracture. I lately saw a man who, at the battle of Gettysburg, had received a Minié ball immediately below the orbit ; the superior maxilary bone was not injured ; the ball followed ihe contour of the face and head, and was extracted posteriorly at the occipital region ; the patient soon recovered.

I shall now say a few words of two of the most frequent and serious complications of gun shot wounds in military hospitals, viz: Erysipelas and hospital gangrene.

I have had the opportunity of observing many cases of both. — As to secondary hemorrhage, another very serious accident after gun shot wounds, I have but seldom observed it. I give here after an account of two of the few cases which came under my observation. Hemorrhage is observed more particularly after incised wounds and this kind of wounds I have but very seldom seen during this war. — In most cases of wounds by conical ball, arteries escape direct injury from them, I have often seen in Italy, as well as during this war, Minié balls traverse the neck *de part en part*, passing through the numerous and important blood vessels of this region, without dividing them. This is probably due to the elasticity, toughness and retractility of the arteries. — But erysipelas and gangrene, the former particularly, have been extremely common. — The pathogeny and treatment of this affection are much better understood to day than they were a few years since. If we consider the circumstances in which it generally occurs and the class of patients it generally affects, we will soon be convinced of the asthenic nature of the disease, we will understand that its apparent symptoms (redness, swelling pains, heat and effusion) which gave rise to the belief, that it was essentially of an inflammatory character, are but the external manifestation of an internal cause — probably a special alteration of the blood. These inflammatory symptoms soon give way to prostration; extensive suppuration soon reduces the strongest man, and sloughing, diarrhœa, delirium follow. Erysipelas affects more partiularly soldiers that have been the most debilitated by privations, hardships and fatigue; it manifests itself in crowded and badly ventilated wards, after severe battles, when the rules of cleanliness are generally neglected. Although frequently idiopathic, it most generally follows wounds and assumes the character of phlegmonous erysipelas; the wound seems to act as an exciting cause, for frequently the simplest incision is followed by erysipelas, when most severe shell and shot wounds do not give rise to it. It is a contagious and infectious disease. A single case of erysipelas introduced in a ward will contaminate the atmosphere, and the disease will very rapidly spread to a large number. — In some cases, cantagion has taken place by means of sponges, bandages and other articles used for dressing wounds. — In consequence, every hygienic precaution should be strictly enforced in a hospital, as soon as a case of erysipelas is declared.

Those affected with this disease should be immediately removed to a distant ward, and preference should always be given to the tents, the great advantages of which I have already mentioned. Plenty of air should be given to the patient in all seasons of the year, and while every prophylactic measure is taken, the proper treatment should be immediately begun. This treatment is another strong argument in favor of the opinion I have expressed concerning the asthœnic nature of the disease.—*Naturam morborum curationes ostendunt.*—If anti phlogistics and abstenious diet are used, the mortality will be very great, experience of late years, but too plainly shows this fact. On the contrary if good nourishment and stimulants are freely given, small will be the number of deaths. We havenow a specific for erysipelas in the tincture of chloride of iron recommended for the first time, a few years ago, by Dr. Bell of Edinburg; it has since been used on a very large scale, and experience has placed its extraordinary efficacity beyond all doubt. I have used it in over 200 cases, with immense benefit; I have often seen it cut short an attack of traumatic erysipelas in 48, 56 hours, and that, without any fear of metastasis on some important organ.

In many cases the tincture of muriate of iron (U. S. Dispensatory) was the only remedy used. It was given in the dose of 10 drops every 2 hours, and in the most serious cases, of 20 in a wine glass of water. The tincture seems to act in improving the condition of the blood, in promotig biliary secretion through its mineral acid, and causing the contraction of the capillaries, thereby relieving congestion and preventing effusion. (Chisolm.)

In erysipelas of the head, accompanied with meningitis or cerebritis, complication which is often observed, we generally prescribed in addition cupping, blisters, etc.— But in many cases of erysipelas extending to a whole limb, and sometimes to the trunk, the Tincture of Iron was the only internal remedy used; in every case, most reliance was placed upon the general treatment. The Tinct. Iron was generally preceded by an active purgative, sometimes by an emetic, when there was much gastric disturbance; in the early inflammatory stage, before suppuration was established; the limb was generally painted with tincture of iodine, or charpie soaked in the solution of sulphate of iron was applied to it. As soon as snppuration is formed, exit must be given to it, by free incisions, and diluted tincture of iodine, Labarraque's solution, or solution of nitrate of silver used to diminish the purulent secretion, and hasten the elimination of sloughs.—The pus, which has such tendency to dissect the tissues, and undermine the skin, should be prevented trom burrowing by properly applied bandages which will in the same time cause the skin to adheres to the deeper parts.

I could give here a very large number of cases, in which the treatment of erysipelas by the tincture of iron has been most successful. But for brevity sake, I will only mention two cases; the first is that of

Mr. Walch, employed in the office of Quarter Master Fisher, who had a most serious attack of erysipelas combined with severe diphtheria; it was during the progress of this disease that crysipelas declared itself, in the face extending very rapidly to the whoie face, ears, scalp and neck, and adding considerably to the dangers of the first already too severe disease. I never saw a more awful case ; the aspect of the patient was really frightful; extensive suppuration took place, and for several days the patient was in a most critical situation,—Repeated cauterisation of the diphtheria pseudo-membranns with muriatic acid and tincture of chloride of iron, given internally; [20 drops every two hours,] with essence of beef, egg-nog and brandy were the principal remedies used. The patient afrer having been in extreme danger, recovered completely.

The other case is that of

G. Smith of Capt. Randolph's Company, employed as courier of Gen. Stonewall Jackson.—This man was wounded at Chancellorsville, on the 3d May 1863, by a Minié ball, cansing compound fracture of the os frontalis. The ball was immediately extracted and the patient was sent to Camp Winder Hospital, at Richmond. One night he ran away from that Hospital, in a state of delirium, and arrived half naked at the Louisiana Hospital. [not far from Camp Winder], where he was received.—At the morning visit, I found him in a serious condition.—The whole head was affected with erysipelas which extended to the neck and anterior part of chest, fever was very high: delirium most violent; the patient could with difficulty be kept in bed; great agitation, pupils very much contracted etc. I immediately prescribed 6 scarified cups at the nape of the neck, followed by sulphat.magnesia cold drinks and a bladder of ice to the head.— In the evening, when the bowels had been thoroughly evacuated, the tinct of muriate of iron was prescribed and continued several days (20 drops every two hours, with purgative enemata, this constituted the treatment, delirium and other acute cerebral symptoms gradually subsided.—On their disappearance nourishment and stimulants given sparingly were administered; the tinct. iron continued at smaller doses.—In the course of 3 days, erysipelas had disappeared, and the patient speedily recovered, his wound healing gradually,

Among the observations at the end will be found an interesting case of erysipelas, invading very nearly the whole body, successfully terminated.

The tincture of iron was almost as useful in hospital gangrene as in erysipelas. The remarks I made concerning the circumstances in which the latter disease originates, are applicable as well to gangrene. The numerous cases I observed occurred in soldiers that had suffered the most, in those of a depraved and infeebled constitution, in whom there was evidently an alteration of the blood. Like erysipelas it is contagious and infectious.— and requires the same hygienic precautions, and above all, the removal of the patients to a pure atmosphere. The treatment in tents was most successful. Burgman reports that hospital gangrene prevailed in one of the low wards at Leyden, whilst the ward or garret above it was free.

The surgeon made an opening in the ceiling between the two, iu order to ventilate the lower or affected ward, and in thirty hours three patients in the upper room, who laid next the opening were attacked by the disease which soon spread through the whole ward. (Chisolm.) In great many cases, the increase or diminution of hospital gangrene was found to correspond with the more or less crowded condition of the wards and the degree of ventilation.—Sponges and other articles when used both for gangrenous and healthy wounds are sure to transmit the disease.

Its principal symptoms are the following: the wound becomes dry, glassy and painful, of a dark gray or ash colour, there is sometimes but a small livid spot in the wound near its circumference. This grayish or darkish slough soon extends to the whole wound, forming a pultaceous and adherent covering, the surrounding surface becomes œdematous, swollen and assumes a livid colour. The discharge is at first diminished in quantity and sanious, but soon becomes profuse, dirty, thick, brownish and highly offensive. It has an odor *sui generis*, which once smelt cannot be forgotten. This discharge is the poison which when applied to a healthy wound, reproduces the terrible disease. The destruction of the tissues is very rapid; in the course of 24 hours, large portions of skin, cellular tissue and muscles are sometimes mortified.

If the phagædenic process is not quickly checked, general symptoms of a serious character soon follow; the pulse loses its strength, becomes feeble and quick; the tongue is dry and brown; diarrhæa, delirium and coma with all the other typhoid symptoms supervene.

Although the local symptoms generally precede the constitutional, these sometimes make their appearance first;—head ache, nausea, perhaps bilious vomiting, hot skin, quick pulse, to which succeed the *local* and other general symptoms. It appears that hospital gangrene may either be a local disease caused by the influence of poisonous matter *sui generis* on the surface of a wound, or a constitutional one caused by the absoption of the poison in the blood.

The most powerful caustics have been used to check the rapid disorganization caused by this disease. Actual cautery is preferred by many French and German surgeons. Guthrie recommends the liberal use of the concentrated mineral acids. My individual experience gives the preference to the pure nitro-muriatic acid. The patient must be placed under the influence of chloroform, and every part of the sore deeply cauterized. I generally used a ball of charpie well impregnated with the acid and caused it to penetrate through all the sinuosities of the wound, and under the neighbouring skin which is generally deeply uudermined. Immediataly after the cauterization, a large carrot poultice (made by scraping raw carrots) is applied to the part. This applicatlon is extremely soothing, absorbs the ichorous discharge, and removes quicker than any thing else the pultaceous sloughs.—I have some times seen the aspect of the wounds change entirely, after a single and well made cauterization followed by the application of the carrot poultice; in some cases, the latter *alone* seems to have been very useful.—

Generally the cauterization must be repeated two or three times.—As I have said before, the patient must be immediately removed to a pure atmosphere, to a tent where he will be alone, in preference. The bowels should be kept free, and the tinct. of iron administered (20 minims every two hours) in conjunction with bark and carbonat-ammonia; brandy and wine, beef-tea, should be given freely.—Opium in repeated doses is of great service to alley the pain, irritability and sleeplessness.—The pain is generally very severe, of a stinging and lancinating character. In many cases it has been alleyed in a very few minutes by the sub cutaneous injection, by the means of Wood's syringe, of a small dose of morphine (1[4 grain in a few drops of water.)

I have found this mode of administering opiates extremely advantageous in a great variety of cases of intense suffering, and generally preferred it to giving morphine by the mouth. In a case of obstinate hiccup, (Lt. Michel of the 14th La), after amputation of leg, which ice and all the anti-spasmodics of the Pharmacopœa had failed to relieve, the repeated injection of small quantities of morphine at the neck, along the course of the pneumogastric nerve, succeeded admirably. I have often seen it relieve immediately most obstinate neuralgia. In cases of local paralysis, the sub cutaneous injection of a very small dose of strychnine (1 1[2 grain) along the nerves, was followed, in many instances, by excellent results.

It is by following the treatment just mentioned, that I have succeeded in a large number of cases to check this frightful disease.

I have already mentioned the case of Michael Quinn, saved from imminent death by removal to an unoccupied and well ventilated room. I could here speak lengthly of several most serious cases in which the treatment was as equally successful. I will only mention the case of Lieut. Errero, of the 10th La, with extensive gangrene of leg (from gun shot wound), penetrating through and through the interoseous space, the patient had suffered besides amputation of the right arm at its superior third; that of private Phelps, of the Washington Artillery, with gun shot wound (Minié) of left arm, followed by Hospital gangrene, which in a few hours extended very rapidly;—this case was very serious, several surgeons had already spoken of amputation. By repeated cauterizations with pure nitro-muriatic acid and the general treatment I have indicated, I succeeded in saving both limb and life; finally the case of sergeant A. Barry of the 9th La. Regt., who had extensive gangrene of the arm, extending to the whole region of the elbow and superior half of fore-arm, the same treatment was followed by excellent results; that of sergt. Dupuis, of the 15th La. Regiment. with gangrene of both legs following shell wounds ; that of J. E. Souby, of the 5th La. Regiment, with gangrene in superior third of thigh, etc., etc.

Pyœmia, or purulent infection, a disease which is so often met with in Europe ;—in the hospitals of Paris it is the chief cause of death after operations,—occurred very rarely in the Louisiana Hospital, and was as rarely observed, I think, in the other hospitals of Richmond.

OBSERVATIONS.

INTERESTING CASE OF RESECTION AT THE ELBOW JOINT.—RECOVERY WITH PERFECT USE OF LIMB.

LIEUT. H. B. MYATT, 26 years old, of the 14th La. Regiment, is wounded on the 27th June 1862, at Gaines Mill, near Richmond, by a Minié ball in the right inguinal region. While being removed on a litter, to the field hospital, he is struck by a random shell, which crushes his left elbow. At the field hospital several surgeons declare that amputation is absolutely necessary. Myatt refuses the operation, and requests to be sent immediately to the Louisiana Hospital of Richmond.

He is admitted on the 28th at 2 o'clock P. M. and we find the following lesions:

1°. Gun shot wound in the right groin.—The ball (Minié) has entered in the internal part, has followed the contour of the femur, internally, and has come out in the posterio-superior part of thigh, without injuring the blood vessels or nerves.—This wound of which there shall be no more question, gave no further trouble.

2°. Considerable ecchymosis at the external and posterior region of left elbow-joint, great swelling, no solution of continuity; comminutive fracture of the two condyles aud olecranon; numerous spiculæ, some of which very sharp, protruding under the skin; the soft tissues of the anterior part of the joint are not much injured.—The patient had previously enjoyed excellent health; he gave us all the particnlars of the accident and said he had opposed amputation on account of his being able to move his fingers; he thought an operation might save his limb.

I immediately proposed the excision of the joint, which was performed that same day in the evening.—The patient being fully under the influence of chloroform, we began the operation.—An incision 5 inches long in the external and posterior region of the elbow, with a small posterior incision falling transversally on the middle of the first, permitted me to operate easily.—All the spiculœ resulting from the crushing of the condyles and olecranon were extracted with the forceps; the flaps were well dissected; the cubital nerve carefully avoided, dissected and pushed aside; the joint was largely opened; the olecranon was sawed off at its base and the humerus resected at two inches above the condyles.—Very little hemorrhage; but one ligature necessary.— The flaps were accurately united by suture, except in the centre, where an exit was left to suppuration. The arm slightly bent was placed a little elevated on a pillow; cold water dressing,—Tincture of arnica and opium mixture.—

June 29th— Moderate reaction.—The patient complains of pains and cramps in the fingers; a little swelling of the hand. A belladona and chloroform liniment is prescribed, and cold irrigation which is continued until the patient leaves his bed. About the fourth day after the operation, suppuration of a healthy character is established and flows freely through the central opening. No accident of any kind; general health continues good; healthy granulations soon begin to form and fill up gradually the enormous cavity. Good nourishment, and brandy twice a day are given to the patient; he takes comp. tinct. of cinchona three times daily.

On the 15th August, the arm was placed slightly bent in a "gouttière" of paste-board, and the tumefaction bandage applied to remove œdema, the patient leaves his bed for the first time. Each time the splint or. -'gouttière" is removed, and the wound dressed, (every 2 or 3 days] passive motions are used to prevent anchylosis.

On the 20th, suppuration has entirely ceased; the wound has closed, and the "gouttière" is dispensed with; the tumefaction bandage is continued on account of persistent œdema of hand.

On the 21st September, Lieut. M. leaves the hospital for the country About the middle of October, he pays us a visit at the hospital, and we perceive with pleasure a continued amelioration. He can bend the forearm on the arm, about one third, hold a fork, a knife or any other small object in that hand; he lifts up a bucket full of water; sensibility and mobility of the fingers are perfect; shortening of the arm is 2 1[2 inches, the left fore-arm and hand are a little atrophied.

On the 30th November Myatt writes: "It seems to me my arm is gaining every day, I can now bend it almost at right angle without the use of the other hand; I can carve my food, tie my cravat, and write a few words with my left hand."

In March 1863, 9 months after the operation, I had the pleasure of seeing again Lieut. Myatt. He then used his left arm with as much facility as the other. Long before the expiration of his leave of absence, he had joined his regiment with which he continued the campaign. At that time there was but little deformity, the excised bones were almost in immediate contact; the size of the pseudo joint was abont normal; in front, its aspect had not changed, and did not indicate that such an operation had been performod. The contractions of the muscles covering the excised bones, were plainly visible; flexion was perfect, and rotation but little impaired; the sensibility of the hand and fingers was intact. I have since that time seen Captain Myatt (he was promoted shortly after his wouud) several times; his health was excellent, and his arm was gaining strength and dexterity every day.

GUN SHOT WOUND OF THE SHOULDER JOINT. RESECTION,—UNSUCCESS.—SECONDARY AMPUTATION.—RECOVERY.

HENRY GRAEL, Company A. 7th La. Regiment, was admitted in the hospital May 9th 1863. He was wounded five days before, at the battle of Frederiksburg by a Minié ball, shattering the superior extremity of the right humerus and causing such lesions as to have necessitated the resection of the upper third of said bone, which was performed on the battle field. The operation was a singular one. There was a triangular flap (letter A) with its apex turned *upwards* and reaching the acromion.

The general health of the patient was good, and the wound had a healthy appearance.

For about six weeks, nothing worth mentioning occurred either in the wound or in the general condition of the patient; nutritious diet and stimulants were given. Two months after the operation, the iucision shad almost entirely healed, when apparently without any cause, the wound assumed a bad aspect; the suppuration became offensive and of an unhealthy character, fever declared itself, and in a day or two, the apex of the flap was mortified: the sloughs were removed and the wound well cauterized with chlorydric acid; Tinct. cinchonœ; tinct of iron, (10 drops every two hours) brandy and egg nog were prescribed. The cauterization was repeated a second time two days after. Under the influence of this active treatment, the wound soon assumed a more healthy appearance; but it continued to secrete a thin and offensive sanies which collecting around the resected extremity of the bone and finding a difficult exit, soon formed several abcesses which were opened. These incisions became fistulous, and the suppuration began to gravitate towards the elbow, causing great swelling and pain, until 3 deep incisions had to be made around the elbow joint. A compressive bandage was applied from the hand upwards, the arm elevated; chloride of Labarraque and tinct. iod. dil. were injected in the fistulous openings; stimulants and tonics administered freely. Still there was no change; the discharge was more and more abundant; the strength of the patient was giving way. Only one of the fistulous openings led to the bone which was found denuded and softened. A long incisiou was made on the external side of the arm with the view of examining the head of the bone, and giving exit to the suppuration which, by pressure around the bone, wonld flow ont abundantly. The bone was found more diseased than I expected, and after a first examination, I was of opinion that nothing, but an amputation, or rather section of the soft parts, the bone being already removed, could save the patient's life.

To this, he refused and reiterated several times hls refusal, until convinced himself, that he was going to die, he consented to the operation which was performed on the 10th August, in very unfavorable circumstances, the patient being extremely debilitated. An ovalar incision was made as for the desarticulation of the shoulder joint—it included the incisions of the first operation—there was but very little loss of blood.—

After the operation, the patient was placed in a tent, was well fed, and had brandy given to him freely; also tinct. bark and iron.

Under this treatment, healthy granulations were soon formed. The patient, though very weak, could not be induced to keep his bed more than three days. At that time, he began to sit up in an arm chair; his appetite became very good; all the functions were regular; 8 days after, the operation, he was walking in the yard and at this date, 3 weeks after, the wound looks very healthy and is healing rapidly.— The humerus examined after the operation was found to be fractured longitudinally and necrosed two inches below the point of section.

SECONDARY AMPUTATION OF HUMERUS.—HEMORRHAGE.—ERYSIPELAS.—SPEEDY RECOVERY.

THOMAS CAVANNAUGH, 22 years of age, private, in Company B. of 15th La. Regiment, [a boatman], was admitted into the hospital on the 9th of October 1862, with compound fracture of humerus received at the battle of Manassas, Augnst 28th 1862. From the date of injnry to the date of admission into hospital, the patient was under treatment at Stanton, where amputation was not deemed necessary; but subsequent injury to the limb from a fall from his bed during a state of intoxication, made it proper in my opinion, that the limb should be sacrificed to save life, and the following lesions as discovered after amputation justified the operation.—Triple fracture extending perpendicularly tc 2 inches above the elbow joint, loose fragments, great infiltration of pus, and sanies in the soft parts, and a collection of same purulent matter in a kind of cupola, formed by the 3 fragments of bone.—Having been an habitual drunkard, his general health was very bad; he was extremely nervous, and exhibited great intolerance to pain; the operation was performed on the 16th; the limb was then amputated by circular method at the apex of the insertion of the deltoid to the humerus—4 interrupted sutures—cold water application' etc. During the night of the third day, after operation, slight hemorrhage ensued, from small artery, which had been simply twisted. It was readily arrested by application of per. chloride of iron. Next morning, erysipelas made its appearance, extending to the axilla and anterior part of chest, immediately combatted by local application of tinct iodine, and internal use of tiuct. mur. ferri, [15 drops every two hours], egg nog and highly nutritons diet, which was continued until the disappearance of all the eresypelatory symptoms; after the subsidence of which, under the use of generous diet and tonics there was rapid improvement,— On the 18th day after amputation, he began to leave his bed, and WAS, on the 25th, day, walking about the hospital, in a fair way, to a speedy and perfect recovery.

TRAUMATIC ANEURISM.— LIGATURE OF BRACHIAL ARTERY.—RECOVERY.

M. J. KENNEDY, 24 years old, private of 6th La. Regiment, Comp. H.. a steamboat man, before enlisting, was wounded on the 29th August 1862, in the middle part of the right arm, by a Minié ball, passing through the soft parts, in the course of the brachial artery. — Very little hemorrhage at the time. The wound healed up in a short time, giving no pain or unusual trouble, On the 30th October, a pulsating tumor was discovered presenting the character of a circumscribed traumatic aneurism; at first very small, it increased gradually in size until it reached that of a hen's egg. The health of the patient was very good, suffering no pain, nor realizing any inconvenience from the tumor. On the 27th January 1863, he entered the hospital.

On the 7th April, the patient being fully under the influence of chloroform, the brachial artery was ligated about one inch above the tumor. At the point of ligation, the artery was easily discovered free from large collateral branches. The state of general health was then very good,— For 72 hours, the heat of the limb was kept up bp sacks filled with warm ashes, cotton wadding, etc. Then the recurrent and anastomotic branches had enlarged sufficiently and increased their action, so as to supply the lower part of the limb with a sufficient circulation,

Pulsations very weak were felt in the aneurism for 48 hours after the operation, but they gradually decreased until the 11th, when they could not be discovered in the sac.

On the 11th, symptoms of erysipelas began to appear around the incision. Local application of solution of sulphate of iron, and tinct. of muriate of iron [10 drops every two hours.]—Opium at night.

April 13th.—Little suppuration of healthy character, erysipelas subsiding; feeble pulsations in the radial artery; good temperature of limb.

April 15th.—Sutures removed; very little suppuration, mostly around the thread; great part of incision has united by first intention. Pulsations of radial artery stronger; none felt in tumor. Cold sensation complained of at end of fingers yesterday, has disappeared to-day.

April 17th.—Very little suppuration; pulsations at wrist not any stronger.—Tumor reduced to half its size.

April 20th.—Pulsations at radial artery increasing; slight tractions on thread.

April 21st.—Thread comes out to-day.

April 22d.—Intermittent and shifting pains on right side of chest, near the median line and numbness of fingers.— Belladona and opium liniment.—Pulsations very good.

April 24th.—Pain and numbness disappeared.—Suppuration entirely ceased.—Full diet.

May 1st.—Use of arm perfect. Tumor appreciable to the touch only.

ERYSIPELAS EXTENDING THE TRUNK, NECK, ARMS AND THIGHS, SUCCESSFULLY TREATED BY THE MURIATIC TINCTURE OF IRON, ETC.

Private G. WALKER, Comp. A. 9th La. Regt., admitted July 18th 1863; wounded at the battle of Gettysburg, by a Minié ball, fracturing left cresta iliaca; the ball remained embedded in the bone, and was extracted.

On admission, the wound had a healthy appearance and the general condition of the patient was good. On the 22d and 25th July, several loose spiculœ were extracted. On the 28th, erysipelas appeared around the wound and gradually spreaded upwards and downwards until the whole abdomen, back and chest were invaded. It there seemed to limit itself. At the first manifestation of the disease, an active purgative was administered, and immediately after Tinct. of Iron was given [20 drops every 2 hours]. An ointment of Sulphate of Iron (1 dragm to 1 ounce of lard] was used morning and night on the whole surface affected with erysipelas. In spite of this treatment, the disease which seemed to have stopped spreading, extended to the neck, arms; and thighs. The fever increased considerably and was accompanied with delirium and great restlesness, soon followed by coma and prostration; there was also some diarrhœa; 2 blisters were applied to inner part of thighs; Carb. of Ammonia, camphor and bark, with astringent enemata prescribed in addition to the Tinct. Iron. In order to check the progress of the erysipelas which threatened to invade every part of the body, a bracelet 1-1|2 inch wide was made by cauterizing with Nitrate of Silver around the fore arms and upper part of legs. —

This treatment seemed to check the disease.

August 25th—The erysipelas did not spread beyond the line of cauterization, and did not invade the head. Consciousness returned; the bowels became more regular, and the patient after having been in a very critical condition, and although now very weak, (August 25th) is gradually but steadily recovering — the wound has a healthy appearance, and discharges but moderately.

GUN SHOT WOUND OF BLADDER — VESSICAL HEMORRHAGE; DEATH.

W. W. RAYNE, aged 19, sergeant 5th La. Co. A. admitted May 9th 1863; wounded on the 30th April at Chancellorsville. The ball went through abdominal parietes a little above Poupart's ligament on the right side aud remains inside. Finger introduced in the wound shows the ball has taken a slanting direction towards the horizontal ramus of the pubis ; two tracks are there felt, one going downwards towards the inside of the thigh, the other towards the bladder. Horizontal ramus of the pubis is fractured and introduction of the finger shows a circular opening through this bone surrounded by sharp spiculœ.

Since reception of injury urine has been constantiy flowing tbrough the wound, patient being unable to void any througb the urethra.

Catheter introduced through urethra in the bladder and there retained; patient laying on his left side, no urine c omes out of wound. As soon as opening of catheter gets blocked up by mucous secretions of the bladder interrupting the flow of urine through it, urine comes ont again through the wound.

Very little fever, — Opium in small doses (gr. 1[4) every 2 hours. Patient sleeps well at night, good appetite. Suppuration from wound on 4th day.

May 13th. small piece of lead found in the opening of catheter, when the instrument is taken out at night.

May 14th, several small spiculœ of bone found in opening of catheter every time it is taken out, urine flowing several times through wound to day on account of those spiculœ blocking up the instrument.

May 15th, extraction of several spiculœ through the wound, 2 of them quite large and angular. Very little loss of blood caused by this extraction.

For several days urine flows well through catheter, all symptoms being good.— May 21st, on extraction of several other spiculœ throngh the wound loss of blood was more abundant than at 1st extraction.

May 24th, irritative fever and hœmorrhage from wound, the blood at first coming out through instrument ; hæmorrhage stopped by application of ice, opium, acetate of lead, etc.,

June 1st, fever and delirium; hæmorrhage again stopped by ice. Acet. of lead and opium continued.

June 2d, pulse quick, small and feeble, delirium, etc. Hæmorrhage, begin in the morning, last all day in spite of iced applications, injection of iced water in the bladder, etc., blood does not coagulate in the bladder, but comes out liquid through instrument. Death during the night of June 4th. Owing to opposition of some of his relations present, no post mortem examination could unfortunately be made.

GUN SHOT WOUND OF FORE ARM;—COMPOUND FRACTURE;—LESION OF RADIAL ARTERY;—REPEATED HEMORRHAGE—AMPUTATION—RECOVERY.

B. D, Herring, age 22, private, Madison artillery, farmer by occupation, is received at the Louisiana Hospital of Richmond, June 4th 1863. The patieut relates that since he has been wounded, May 4th 1863, hemorrhage has been occurring from his wound every 4 or 5 days; it was stopped each time either by the application of a "tourniquet" around the arm or by styptics. He is admitted with a "tourniquet" around the arm. A Minié ball entered his left fore arm on the inside at the junction of the lower and middle third, and came out on the outside a little above the wound of entrance, denuding the cubitus and causing comminutive fracture of radius and severing the radial artery

The "tourniquet" being removed, blood comes out abundantly, but not in jet, from the wound; the latter being cleared from coagula and spiculœ, blood is seen oozing from the distal side of the radial artery; the patient was exausted by repeated loss of blood and very pale.

June 5th, the patient being under the influence of chloroform, the circular amputation of fore arm was performed at the union of the middle and upper third; but very little loss of blood. — Tincture of iron and bark with brandy. were given freely — reunion took place by granulations without a single bad symptom.

On the 30th June, the patient was furloughed, the wound being entirely united, except in a small point in the centre.

GUN SHOT WOUND OF THE HEAD; LOSS OF BOTH EYES—RECOVERY.

C. Davenport, 21 years old, Compary H., 2d La Regiment, admitted in the hospital May the 9th 1863. Wounded May 3d at Chancellorsville by a Minié ball entering external canthus of right eye, and coming out horizontally about one inch back of left temporal ridge, passing through the ethmoid. The eye lids on both sides are closed, red and swollen; on examination both eyes are found completely destroyed, the orbital cavities are filled with sloughs, no signs of the tissues of the eye. Patient very much depressed and feeble; Cough incessant caused by blood running into the throat; this blood mixed with mucous secretions is coughed out with a very large quantity of small spiculæ.

Spiculæ come out also through opening of exit; with very few exceptions, they are all exceedingly small, almost like dust. No appetite, no fever, no pains in the head. Prescription: Tinct. Cinchon. composit, and mustard foot bath at night. Some diarrhæ about the 5th day; restlessness. Chalk mixture; small doses of sulphate of morphine at night

May 20th; no more cough; [blood and spiculæ] cease to run into the throat. Wound of exit becomes fistulous. General health good. The patient gets out of bed; steady improvement. The two orbital cavities are hidden by the eye lids, of which the left is prominent as if the eye ball was still remaining; the linings of the cavities are also of a red natural healthy colour; the mucous membrane of the superior eyelid is irritated by the eye lashes of the inferior. The principal interest of the case consists in this, that no symptoms of disorder of the brain have ever manifested themselves,

A furlough was granted the patient on the 11th June; he left the hospital in care of a friend, in very good health.

GUN SHOT WOUND ON BOTH THIGHS.—PROFUSE HEMORRHAGE.—RECOVERY.

E. N. Butler, (private), aged 21, Co. A., 30th N. C. Reg., admitted

May 9th 1863.—Wounded May 3rd by a Minié ball, passing through both thighs, at upper part of lower third, without injury to the bone. The wounds were progressing favorably and healing until the 21st May. During that night, a profuse hemorrhage from the right thigh took place Before the assistant surgeon on duty could arrive, the mattress was soaked through half its thickness, pulse hardly perceptible, no conciousness and involuntary passage from the bowels. Pressure on femoral artery for a few minutes, stopped the hemorrhage. Injection of per chloride of iron and charpie, impregnated with same introduced in the wound. Opium pills of 1[2 grain given every three hours, and Tinct, Muriat of Iron 10 drops every hour.

The day after, conciousness hardly recovered. By degrees, with small doses of opium and continuation of Tinct Iron and stimulants given sparingly, the patient recovered. Suppuration loosens the charpie 6 days after the hemorrhage, which was not renewed.

The patient was furlouged on the 12th June still weak but in good health, the wounds were closed.

A TREATISE ON GUN-SHOT WOUNDS

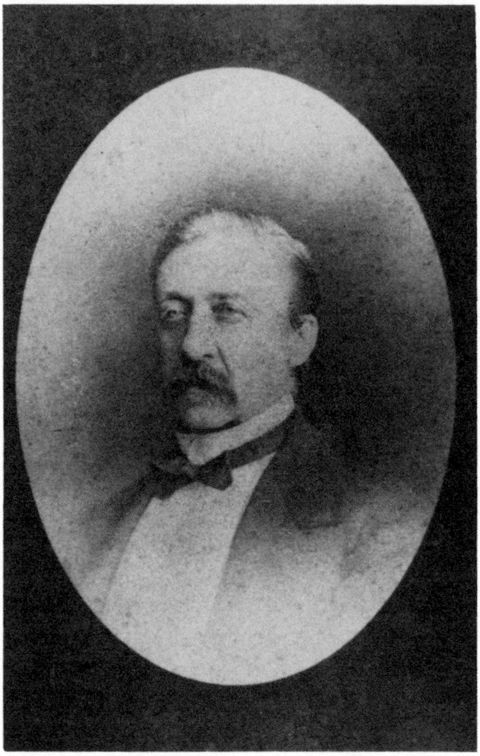

Moritz Schuppert

1817–1887

Portrait Collection, Rudolph Matas Medical Library

Tulane University

Moritz Schuppert

Moritz Schuppert was born in Marburg, Germany, in 1817. Little information is available about his early years, although it is known that his family was relatively affluent. Accordingly, he is stated to have received a classical education, including medical school. Following graduation, he married and, after completing post-graduate training, decided to emigrate to the United States.

The year in which Schuppert arrived in America remains unknown, but he did settle in New Orleans in the early 1850s. This final move must have been part of his original intent in coming to the United States because in the mid-nineteenth century many German-speaking physicians, drawn by a growing German population, were establishing themselves in Louisiana. Unfortunately, the divergent medical backgrounds of these immigrant physicians, combined with their nationalistic fervor, created antagonisms between them and their English- and French-speaking peers.

On arrival in New Orleans Schuppert had few friends and little knowledge of English. However, in the course of time his medical training and surgical skills became apparent. In 1853, he was appointed a visiting surgeon to the Charity Hospital and also participated in the care of numerous patients during a particularly severe yellow fever epidemic. Perhaps as a result of this experience, many of the articles that he eventually contributed to medical journals dealt with quarantine practices and the etiology of yellow fever. Schuppert was named city physician in 1854.

Five years later, he established, with Samuel Choppin (1828–1880), the Orthopaedic Institution located on Carondelet Street. Although named "Orthopaedic," the facility was in fact a private hospital meant to treat "all deformities of the body, both congenital and acquired, such as club foot, club-hand, wry-neck, distortions of the spine, of joints, anchylosis, dislocations, contractions from burns, wounds, etc.; with special attention to the radical cure of hernia, and also to the treatment of the diseases of the genito-urinary organs."

Through hard work Schuppert became one of the most distinguished surgeons of New Orleans. He is known to have performed considerable numbers of surgical operations, and was especially skilled in the treatment of orthopedic deformities.

Detailed records of Schuppert's service during the Civil War are not available. Because of his age, he probably did not see much active battlefield service, but instead continued to practice and treat the wounded in New Orleans. Schuppert's *Treatise on Gun-shot Wounds* was originally published in the *New Orleans Medical and Surgical Journal,* where most of his writings initially appeared.

In early May 1869, the American Medical Association for the first time held its annual meeting in New Orleans. Among the Louisiana physicians who played a prominent role in that gathering was Schuppert, who read a lengthy paper concerning operations for vesico-vaginal fistula. Although he was later involved in many non-surgical aspects of medicine, Schuppert was always known for his prodigious surgical feats, including one of the earliest excisions of a scapula with preservation of a useful arm.

Perhaps Schuppert's most lasting contribution to Southern surgery was the introduction of the concept of Listerism into that region of the United States. He continued to monitor German medical literature after leaving Germany and, having read about the remarkable results achieved with the Listerian technique, decided in 1875 to visit Europe and learn about the new method firsthand. He returned to America in the fall of 1875 after having spent the summer months traveling through Europe and promptly became a major proponent of Lister's technique. He soon authored an important article reporting the results of antiseptic treatment of wounds in German hospitals and explaining the theory of septic infection. This remains one of the earliest papers in American surgical practice devoted to the results of Lister's antiseptic methods.

Although Schuppert's articles on Listerism met with skepticism and even hostility from his colleagues, he remained fully committed to his beliefs. This was most evident in his surgical wards at the Charity Hospital. Despite other physicians' protests, Schuppert immediately began to utilize Lister's techniques, and by January 1878 he had performed over 120 "antiseptic" operations. Based on this experience he wrote a second article on the antiseptic treatment of wounds in 1878. In all, Schuppert's operations had only a four percent mortality, an unbelieveably low figure for that era. It should be noted that none of these operations was on the abdomen, but it was the rare surgeon who ever performed abdominal surgery during those years.

Schuppert constantly stressed the fact that it was mandatory to follow the Lister method completely, without omitting or altering a single aspect. Most important, he emphasized the need for disinfecting any object that came into contact with a wound with a 3 percent carbolic acid water solution.

Despite Schuppert's championing of Lister's methods, the concept of antiseptic surgery made as slow a progress in Louisiana as anywhere else in the country. Unfortunately, Schuppert's methods were immediately discontinued following his retirement from the Charity Hospital, and were not to be reintroduced until 1887 after a severe outbreak of puerperal fever in the obstetrical wards.

Schuppert was also involved in a fierce debate regarding vaccination and bloodletting. In the middle of the nineteenth century, New Orleans suffered from a series of smallpox epidemics, which were the occasion of public outcry over the need for compulsory vaccination and effective quarantine measures. Although most opposition to these efforts was concentrated among the uneducated, a number of prominent citizens, including physicians, continuously criticized any attempts at prevention. Schuppert was perhaps the most influential and outspoken member of this opposition group. In November 1879, in an article in the *New Orleans Medical and Surgical Journal* he bitterly attacked the practice of vaccination, arguing that it was against all principles of common sense. Schuppert denied the existence of cowpox and quoted statistics to attempt to prove that vaccination was useless in preventing smallpox. Further, Schuppert even charged that vaccination had been previously responsible for transmitting syphilis and other contagious diseases.

In October 1882, he appealed to his profession in an article for a return to the use of bloodletting. He wrote that the continued use of the lancet was essential for treatment of many ailments, including eclampsia, congestive and inflammatory diseases of internal organs, wounds involving the peritoneum, and traumatic injuries to the brain and other viscera.

Although few details are available concerning Schuppert's family, it is known that his own children were seriously infected with smallpox during one of the many epidemics. Two of his sons, Charles and William, became physicians and assisted their father during numerous operations.

Despite his talents, Schuppert was in many ways limited by a difficult personality and by parochial thinking. An obituary in the *New Orleans Medical and Surgical Journal* noted that he was thought of as "a man of rugged individuality, of strong prejudices, of bitter hates, of deep-rooted convictions, which he would have dared maintain against the world. Through all his long life he knew the unutterable sorrow of hiding beneath an abrupt and repellant manner and a stern exterior." Schuppert died on May 2, 1887.

A TREATISE

ON

GUN-SHOT WOUNDS:

WRITTEN FOR AND DEDICATED TO THE

Surgeons of the Confederate States Army,

BY

M. SCHUPPERT, M. D.,

Of New Orleans, Louisiana.

NEW ORLEANS:

PRINTED AT THE BULLETIN BOOK AND JOB OFFICE.

1861.

CONTENTS.

Part I.

Gun-Shot Wounds.

PAGE.

General Observations.—Provisional Bandages.—Transportation of the wounded.—Management of Military Hospitals.... 5

Injuries to the Shaft of Bones:

Nature of Injuries.......... 8
Diagnosis.......... 11
Prognosis.......... 12
Treatment.......... 12

Injuries to the Joints:

Nature of Injuries.......... 21
Prognosis.......... 22
Diagnosis.......... 24
Treatment.......... 24

Part II.

Injuries to the Single Bones—Upper Extremity.

Humerus.......... 27
Shoulder-Joint.......... 28
Elbow-Joint.......... 32
Fore-Arm.......... 36
Wrist.......... 37
Hand.......... 37

Lower Extremity.

Femur.......... 38
Hip-Joint.......... 40
Knee-Joint.......... 43
Leg.......... 44
Foot.......... 45

Gun-Shot Wounds of the Body.

Wounds of the Body.......... 46

A TREATISE

ON

GUN-SHOT WOUNDS:

WRITTEN FOR AND DEDICATED TO THE

Surgeons of the Confederate States Army,

BY

M. SCHUPPERT, M. D.,

Of New Orleans, Louisiana.

NEW ORLEANS:

PRINTED AT THE BULLETIN BOOK AND JOB OFFICE.

1861.

PREFACE.

We are in the midst of a Revolution in which Southern rights and Southern chivalry are arrayed against Northern aggression and Northern fanaticism. Large armies are rushing to the contest, and while preparing for the deadly struggle, all the appliances of modern warfare will be brought in requisition. We may, therefore, expect to see many a bloody battle, many a hard won field. The soldier is already dreaming of glory and renown, and, therefore, eagerly grasps the theories of war; but military tactics necessarily leave out of the question the ghastly field, its wounded, and the bed of suffering. There the province of the physician begins, and on the field of battle itself, his knowledge and skill are put to the severest test. He must be prepared and ready for every emergency; he has no time to consult, no time to read up, he must act; for while he hesitates, the current of life may be ebbing away. We have thought that a short manual on the treatment of gun-shot wounds might be serviceable at the present time, and though we admit that many are more competent for the task, none will undertake it with more zeal.

INTRODUCTION

In the following pages we propose to present our readers with a brief and practical account of the treatment of gun-shot wounds. While omitting all theoretical discussions, we intend to explain principally the treatment of those gun-shot wounds which are complicated with injuries of the bones. Our views and treatment are based upon the experience of some of the most celebrated military surgeons of the age, and that experience is gained by a treatment of over two thousand shot-wounds, in the late war in Schleswig-Holstein.* Boldly may we assert, says Esmarch, that those three years' experience in the treatment of gun-shot wounds has established a new era in the history of military surgery. It is now settled beyond a doubt, that in future, amputations will not be deemed indispensable, and that, though primary resections of the shaft of bones are generally to be considered a dangerous enterprise, resections in joints are a new and great acquisition. More than three hundred doctors from all parts of Germany, have witnessed the favorable results chiefly obtained from resections of the elbow-joint. The prejudice of old military surgeons, who thought that resection of a joint was inadmissible during war, must now be done away with, for experience has shown that this operation was successful under circumstances where even amputation proved fatal.

* We have derived the greatest information in this respect from the invaluable writings of Stromeyer, Surgeon-in-Chief, and Esmarch, Physician to the Staff, in the army of Schleswig-Holstein.

TREATISE ON GUN-SHOT WOUNDS.

GENERAL OBSERVATIONS.--PROVISIONAL BANDAGES.--TRANSPORTATION OF THE WOUNDED.--MANAGEMENT OF MILITARY HOSPITALS.

Capital operations are seldom executed on or near the battle field; yet it is well known that when amputation of an injured limb is indicated, every hour's delay diminishes the chance of the patient's recovery. In most cases the wounded are conveyed to the hospitals with a temporary bandage. It is here that we experience the most painful disappointments. Operations however skillfully executed, very seldom result favorably, notwithstanding the most careful after-treatment. The principal cause of this frightful mortality is mismanagement of the wounded on the field of action, together with the miserable conveyances on which the wounded are usually carried, sometimes over a distance of many miles to some hospital. Thus it is that a crushing of any one of the long bones is soon followed by the symptoms of concussion in the whole limb; all the cellular tissues around the wound, including the nerves and vessels, are covered with extravasated blood, sensitiveness is diminished from the shock and compression of the nerves, causing a kind of paralysis. The circulation in the veins is diminished, and this stasis of blood is soon followed by an abundant exudation of serum, infiltrating all the soft parts. The wounded are conveyed from the field of battle on badly constructed wagons, which cause them to suffer excruciating pain; the muscles of the injured limb become spasmodically contracted, so that the fragments of the splintered bone are driven into the flesh. We frequently find, moreover, that ill adjusted bandages increase the evil. From fear of hemorrhage, the surgeon applies a roller around the injured limb. This bandage being put on tightly, acts as a tourniquet, stops the circulation, but increases the serous exudation; should there happen to be a laceration of one of the larger blood-vessels, the bandage increases the danger, for the blood, though prevented from escaping externally, becomes infiltrated into the cellular tissue; the pressure and swelling which are thereby occasioned, being generally followed by gangrene of the whole extremity. The care, says Esmarch, with which the wounded were properly bandaged and conveyed from the battle field to the hospitals, was probably the means of bringing about the happy results which followed the subsequent treatment of many severe injuries, complicated with lesions of the bone, after the battle of Idstedt. The surgeon who accompanies the army on the field of battle has, therefore, great responsibility; for, upon his preliminary dressing much of the result of the after treatment depends. It ought to be his chief aim to support the wounded limb in such a way that the fragments of the bones cannot be displaced during transportation, and also, that the sufferer be made as comfortable as possible. For this purpose, a well applied bandage, with splints, resting on a pillow stuffed with finely cut straw or oat-chaff, will prove very servicable.

In fractures of the humerus, the best bandage that can be used is a small cushion placed between the chest and the fractured limb, the latter of course being supported by a mitella (sling) and a roller around the body.

A fractured thigh should be placed in an abducted position and rotated outwards, supported on a large pillow filled with chaff, or placed on a double inclined plane. A fractured leg is best attended to by putting it in a fracture box, which consists of four boards—a bottom, two sides, and a foot board, joined by hinges, in such a way that they can close at right angles, and thus receive the wounded limb properly supported on a pillow.

A fractured forearm should be placed on a properly padded

splint, care being taken not to exercise undue pressure on the internal condyle.

The wagons used for transporting the wounded should have good springs. In default of these, moveable springs could easily be provided so as to be adapted to the interior of any wagon. On these springs a light frame work can rest, to receive a mattrass upon which the wounded can lie.

As soon as the wounded arrive at the hospital, it is the duty of the surgeon in attendance, to make at once a careful examination of the wounds. This examination is of the utmost importance, for it has to decide whether an operation is necessary or not. If the injury is found to be of such a nature that an attempt to save the limb would hazard the life of the patient, amputation must be performed at once. The advantage of immediate action is acknowledged by all military surgeons. On the other hand, in attempting to save the injured limb, great care should be taken to maintain a perfect adaptation of the fragments of bone together. The simplest apparatus are always the best. We have already mentioned cushions filled with oat-chaff as very advantageous in this respect. The surgeon should not leave the bed of his patient until he has placed him in such a position as to relieve him from all pain. Laborious and tiresome as this may be, the good results which the surgeon obtains, are, besides the thanks of the sufferer, sufficient compensation for the trouble.

Another important point in the treatment of the wounded, is the selection of proper places for the establishment of hospitals. Buildings should be well ventilated in order to prevent the development of miasma. Such localities, therefore, ought to be selected, which admit of a plentiful supply of fresh air. Unfortunately, it often happens after a battle, that the wounded must be placed in localities which are unfit for hospital purposes: still the surgeon can do much in such cases towards improving the condition of his patients by attention to ventilation. He should not fear a draft of air as much as a deficiency in this respect. The war of Schleswig-Holstein has proved that the best results were obtained in those localities where a permanent ventilation was instituted day and night.

As the surgeon will meet with prejudice from the wounded and the nurses; it may become necessary to have the window-shutters permanently removed, so that the regulations may be certainly carried out. Cleanliness is of the utmost importance in a hospital. In dressing the wounded, also, too much cleanliness cannot be used. The dressings soaked with pus and blood should be taken out of the room immediately after being removed from the patient. Sponges should not be used at all, as it is impossible to keep a separate sponge for each patient. The wounds should be first washed with warm water poured out from a spout and afterward wiped with dry charpie.

INJURIES TO THE SHAFT OF BONES.

THE NATURE OF THOSE INJURIES.

In a critical examination of gun-shot wounds of the long bones, we must make a distinction between those which injure the continuity or shaft of the bone, from those which implicate the joints or the extremity of the bones. For injuries of the joints involve more dangerous consequences than injuries in the length of a bone. Before taking up this subject, however, we shall say a word in regard to the injuries caused by cannon-shot or bomb-shells. Wounds from such projectiles are generally accompanied with extensive laceration of the soft parts, or loss of the entire limb. Such wounds generally prove fatal, on account of the shock to the nervous system; death commonly taking place in the first twenty-four hours, or mortification may ensue from which the patient dies usually by the fourth day. The loss of an arm does not necessarily prove fatal, but the danger increases with the proximity of the injury to the trunk. For we often find simultaneous injuries of internal organs, as for instance, rupture of the liver and spleen. Not less dangerous are those injuries where extensive fractures of the bones have taken place, though the soft parts are uninjured. We diagnose the frightful extent of such injuries by the singular sensation derived from the crepitation of the fragments of bone when we press upon the limb. Mortification here commonly ensues. The only chance of recovery in such cases is to amputate at once so as to save the wounded the pain of transportation, for this is certain death.

When a ball strikes the shaft of a bone at right angles, going through a limb, the bone is generally shivered into many fragments. The size and number of these splinters vary considerably, many of them being still connected with the soft parts. It is now well settled by a great number of observations, that these fragments retain their vitality, as long as the periosteum is not detached from the surrounding parts, and that they can be united by callus to their fragments.

Baudens, in his "Clinique des plaies d'armes à feu," adopts Dupuytren's classification of splinters into primary, secondary and tertiary, and recommends the extraction of all splinters, whether loose or still connected with the integuments; and he further advances the principle, that all bones should be resected as far as a fissure exists; but experience has proved that this precept is dangerous. Fissures, like splinters, may heal by the formation of callus. The older surgeons regarded fissures as very dangerous, an opinion which has some foundation, if inflammation and putrefaction should happen to supervene; for then necrosis will follow, unless the patient should succumb from phlebitis, a complication which is very frequent in wounds associated with fractured bones. The danger increases when the fissure extends into the joint. But, as in fractures of the bones of the skull, at least in young individuals, a fissure seldom extends beyond one bone, on account of the sutures, the same thing takes place in the long bones. There fissures of the shaft seldom reach the joint, neither will a ball passing through the epiphysis cause a fissure of the shaft. It is only when a ball happens to strike the exact point of union between these two parts, that a fissure may extend in both directions. The explanation of this fact is easily found, if we bear in mind that the shaft and extremities of bones are formed by separate points of ossification, and do not unite until a mature age, being, however, connected by cartilaginous tissue. In the war of Schleswig-Holstein, fractures combined with splinters and extensive fissures were frequently seen in the tibia. If the fibula be not implicated, the full extent of the injury may escape detection. The surgeon in such a case removes the loose splinters, and endeavors to save the limb; but generally, however appropriate the treatment otherwise may be, extensive inflammation and suppuration will set in. Some cases recover after the removal of large splinters which were either loose in the first place, or became so by necrosis. In other instances, secondary bleeding takes place during the suppurative process to such an extent as to require amputation, though the life of the patient will seldom be saved by it.

If the ball have lost some of its projectile power, it may cause a simple fracture, and the ball itself be found between the fractured ends or near them in the soft parts. It may happen that the clothes be not perforated, and the place where the ball struck be driven into the wound, and then some movement of the patient or pulling on the clothes might have brought out the ball, though the patient be not aware of it. It is therefore important to examine attentively the wearing apparel of the patient.

A simple fracture may again be caused though the ball retain its full force, if it happen to hit the bone obliquely instead of a right angle. In such cases the ball, after touching the bone, glances in another direction, so that a straight line from the place by which the ball entered to that of its exit would seem to leave the bone untouched. On probing the wound with the fingers, the fracture will be at once detected. In such cases a proper treatment, under favorable circumstances, will generally preserve the limb. We have seen, says Esmarch, a great number of such injuries of the thigh-bone recover perfectly; the prognosis being unfavorable only in such cases where the fracture was near the upper third of the femur or in the trochanter itself.

It frequently happens that a portion of the shaft of a bone

may be shot off without fracturing the bone itself. These cases generally have a favorable result. On the other hand, a ball may penetrate the bone, remain in it or pass through it without the bone being fractured or splintered. Such cases, which occur mostly in the upper portion of the tibia, allow a favorable prognosis. Finally, a ball may strike a bone and become flattened against it, without causing a fracture. But those portions of the bone which are struck, generally mortify, for the periosteum is necessarily destroyed. Such cases, where one of the long bones has been so injured, when brought into over-crowded hospitals, are apt to cause suppuration of the medulla, and death commonly follows by purulent absorption.

EXAMINATION OF THE WOUNDS.

No task appears easier than to recognize an injury of a bone if accompanied by an external wound. For such injuries, it seems, could be more closely examined than simple uncomplicated fractures; experience proves, nevertheless, that error occurs more often than the correct diagnosis. This can be explained by the abuse which the surgeons generally make of their probes, for they commonly use this instrument in their examination, though in reality nothing can be learned from it, whereas the finger is the best and most reliable probe. It would be well, says Stromeyer, if all the probes could be confiscated at the beginning of a war, for then surgeons would have to use their fingers instead. Another difficulty in the examination of gun-shot wounds arises from their very nature. Whereas in ordinary fractures the periosteum is generally separated with the bone, in gun-shot wounds the periosteum may remain entire, though the bone itself is fractured, so that the form and position of the bone remain apparently intact. This deception will occur even after a digital examination, if the limb be not examined in the same position in which it was when the injury occurred. The deeper the wound, the more difficult the diagnosis becomes. In this condition, if a doubt arises as to sacrificing or preserving the limb, and a digital examination cannot settle the question, the surgeon should not hesitate to make a free incision so as to increase the original wound, in order to examine its exact condition.

PROGNOSIS.

There is no doubt that a gun-shot wound complicated with an injury of the bone, is more dangerous than without it. The gravity of the injury is proportioned to the size of the bone, and the prognosis rendered more doubtful the nearer the wound approaches the trunk. The condition of the soft parts, which are generally lacerated by the fractured bone, exercise a great influence upon the extent and gravity of the subsequent inflammation. That the fracture itself does not aggravate the case, is easily demonstrated by comparing the result of those cases where only one bone was broken, with those in which both were fractured. The former generally progress favorably and the inflammation is circumscribed; but when the fragments of the bone have been displaced by the action of the muscles, keeping up a constant irritation, as occurs when both bones are broken, then the most extensive inflammation will be found. Another serious consideration in the prognosis of these injuries is their tendency to pyæmia, a circumstance which might be explained by the anatomical fact, that the veins of bones are always open, having no power of contractility, and therefore greatly favor the absorption of pus. It is of the utmost importance to find means by which the medulla of a long bone could be protected against purulent absorption. Certain constitutions are not susceptible of pyæmic intoxication; nevertheless, many of these sink from the exhaustion which accompanies an extensive suppurating wound.

TREATMENT.

A fresh wound is not aggravated by introducing the finger, to ascertain the extent of the injury, or to remove foreign substances, such as the ball or pieces of cloth together with the fragments of bone which are detached. When it is required to enlarge a wound it should be done in the line of the long axis of the bone.

When the ball can be easily felt by the finger, a strong forceps should be introduced, guided by the index finger of the left hand, and as soon as the forceps touches the ball, the finger is withdrawn, the ball seized with the forceps and extracted. We must carefully abstain from too long a search for a ball, and if it cannot be easily reached, or cut out on the opposite side, it should be left untouched. Of all foreign substances, a bullet is the most harmless, as proved by numerous instances in which it has remained in the bones. What is true of the ball, is also applicable to splinters. Those which are entirely separated from the bone, should alone be removed. It is remarkable, how frequetly fractures heal after a small exfoliation of bone, when no attempt was made to extract any splinter. This generally occurs, where the ball having passed entirely through the limb, and where there was no necessity to search for the projectile. Those splinters which are still connected with the periosteum should be the last removed ; even if the periosteum be separated from the bone during the subsequent inflammatory process it will assist in the formation of a new bone, whereas, in the beginning a splinter could not be removed without carrying with it the periosteum. On the principle above stated, remarks Stromeyer, I consider extensive resections in the continuity of bones inadmissible in recent wounds, because they cannot be executed without simultaneous removal of the periosteum, for then the ends of the bone are less apt to unite, than when this membrane is intact. Besides this, a resection of bone increases the liability of inflammation or suppuration. I do not wish, however, to be understood as arguing against sawing off the sharp and pointed fragments of bone, if it can be done without enlarging the wound. All the cases in which extensive resections were performed during the campaign invariably proved fatal. The precautions which are necessary even for the extraction of foreign substances in wounds of recent date, are still more necessary when the opening made by the ball is so swollen, that the finger can hardly enter without causing the patient great pain. In such cases an examination ought only to be made when an operation is dependent upon the diagnosis. If there be any hope of preserving the limb, the wound should not be touched, either with the finger or probe. In fresh wounds an incision may be sometimes indicated, to get rid of a quantity of extravasated blood collected near the fracture, but after an interval of twenty-four hours, such an incision is entirely inadmissible, for it would allow the entrance of air to the collected blood, would cause it to decompose, and thereby prevent its absorption; it also increases inflammation and suppuration, and therefore the tendency to necrosis in the fractured ends of the bone. On the contrary, when inflammation can be subdued, we find that the splinters which are already loose will alone be separated, and only the ends of the fractured bones exfoliated. Knowing the obnoxious influence of a necrosed bone in retarding the healing process of a wound, it should be our greatest care to remove this source of irritation. But this is not always in the power of the surgeon. The great means of preventing inflammation and necrosis, are, *rest, antiphlogistic treatment, and free discharge of pus.* If the prognosis be favorable, and hope of preserving the injured limb be entertained, the attending surgeon should place the wounded extremity in such a manner that the fragments of bone cannot be displaced and irritate the surrounding muscles. Large cushions filled with chaff or chopped straw will be of the greatest advantage. If the extremity be shortened by a displacement of the ends of the fractured bone, no attempt should be made to overcome the deformity by any method of traction, for some time after the patient has been admitted into the hospital. The consequence of such an attempt would only produce fresh irritation of the soft parts without the end being accomplished. On the other hand, a few days' rest, under a proper treatment, will result in a relaxation of the muscles, and then the bones can be easily brought in a better position and retained there by splints. The treatment of wounds should be as simple as possible. The leading principle for the surgeon is to watch closely the condition of the wound, and remove all influences which interfere with the healing process. When wounded men were brought to the hospitals, says Esmarch, with the shafts of the long bones crushed by balls, if the limbs were already well bandaged and supported by splints on the field of battle, and the external appearance did not indicate infiltration or some other dangerous complication, we let them remain as they were. After placing the limb properly, cold applications were used, and no attempt made to remove splinters, or interfere with the wound in any other way. Under such a treatment we have seen cases recover in a short time, with very little suppuration, even where the thigh-bone itself was fractured. The wounded limb should be brought, if possible, into such a position, that it can be dressed without being moved. The greatest injury that can be done to a wounded limb in the beginning of the treatment, is to move it too often. The importance of keeping a wounded limb completely at rest, is unfortunately not so generally understood as it ought to be. This will spare the patient much pain, and avoid slight and repeated bleeding,—together with irritation which keeps up inflammation.

Another element in the proper management of gun-shot wounds, consists in an antiphlogistic treatment. That great man, John Hunter, says in his treatise on gun-shot wounds, that the injuries of the extremities did not bear blood-letting as well as injuries of the trunk. This doctrine is approved by most surgeons says Stromeyer, but, as I have already stated in relation to the treatment of simple fractures, I consider it erroneous, and have always seen the best results follow venesection in the treatment of complicated gun-shot wounds. But, alas ! the value of blood-letting, is like so many other valuable remedies, now discredited, and expectant homœopathy seems to rule the day, so that young physicians are afraid to practice venesection. As they treat pneumonia, without blood-letting they think it just as reasonable to avoid venesection in traumatic injuries of the body. The small and contracted pulse, which is so commonly met with in recent gun-shot wounds, seems to forbid venesection, but in most cases such a pulse will be found to rise soon after blood-letting. The appropriate time for bleeding is within the first three days after the patient recovers from the first shock.

If suppuration has taken place, venesection is no longer indicated, though leeches may still be sometimes used with advantage, when applied in the neighborhood of the fracture to diminish the inflammatory swelling; they will dispense with incisions, which otherwise may be required. When suppuration sets in *slowly*, venesection may be performed even after the third day, with benefit to the patient.

Many surgeons are averse to blood-letting in complicated fractures, because they fear to weaken the patient in anticipation of the suppurative process which commonly follows these injuries; but these surgeons do not consider that suppuration will be diminished in proportion as the inflammatory process is shortened. I have seen several patients die delirious within four days, from injuries of the upper extremities, from too much inflammation, and I am convinced that blood-letting would have prevented it. Younger surgeons, therefore, should not be afraid of drawing blood; and this was the practice of the English surgeons during the French war, a practice which we entirely approve. Although the type of disease of our times appears to be less inflammatory than thirty years ago, and although practical surgery is bound to profit by the lessons of internal pathology, we think, nevertheless, that a mechanical lesion, such as a gun-shot wound, must be treated on different principles than a case of pneumonia, pleurisy, or typhoid fever.

Next to blood letting, cold applications, the use of ice, cold irrigations are the most efficacious remedies. The principal action of these cold water applications is to keep down inflammation and prevent early suppuration. These means will also facilitate the absorption of much of the extravasated blood, between and near the fractured parts of bone. If no care be taken to diminish inflammation and suppuration, the extravasated blood is turned into pus; which, added to the swollen and inflamed parts will exercise an undue pressure upon the veins, and by interfering with the circulation of the blood, will cause a stagnation and serous infiltration of the whole limb. This condition is often a precursory symptom of phlebitis and death. It seldom occurs in hospitals where iced applications have been made early. In using cold applications, it is necessary to make them directly on the wound. Charpie and sticking plasters should be avoided, as they prevent a free discharge from the wound. Another mistake is to cover the cold applications with oiled silk, for, by preventing evaporation, it causes the dressings to get warm sooner, requiring fresh applications of cold, and these too frequent alternations of heat and cold irritate the parts and increase congestion. The antiphlogistic treatment described above, accompanied by a low diet and mild saline purgatives, will be found the best. Cold applications should be continued as long as they prove agreeable to the patient. In wounds of the joints, we have seen ice applied during six or eight weeks with the best result.

If these cold applications should not be tolerated any further by the patient, they ought to be replaced by poultices, or perhaps by warm water dressings. The latter, while they fulfil all the effects of a poultice, are preferable: they are easier removed, they are cleaner, and the patient can apply them himself, thus dispensing with the constant services of a nurse, an object of some importance in crowded wards. In wounds situated near the extremities of the forearm and legs, if the bones are much injured and many small splinters exist, then warm poultices or better still, warm water baths, will be found exceedingly beneficial. They relax the tension of the parts, promote the discharge of pus, and act favorably on the capillary vessels on the surface of the limb. For this purpose, tin boxes eight inches high, of the same width, and two feet long, having a lid, and an opening at the end for the reception of the limb, will answer very well. They are to be filled with warm water, which might be kept warm for a longer period by means of blankets.

Finally, an important point in the management of the wounds is a free discharge of pus, besides the protection of the limb from serous infiltration. For serous exudation, if allowed to collect, will soon be replaced by pus; whereas this will not be the case when a proper opening is made to facilitate the discharge of all fluids. The best proof hereof, is found in the treatment of the parts situated beneath the deep facia. If incisions be made early, when exudations are simply serous, the suppuration will be found to diminish ; but if incisions are not made early, extensive suppuration will follow, impeding the treatment, and endangering the life of the patient. This is especially true of gun-shot wounds. Sometimes a ball after striking a bone glances in a different direction, lacerating the muscles, and burrowing beneath the fascia, so that the finger cannot ascertain the direction of the ball. In such cases pus accumulates in these sinuses, as it cannot escape by the narrow and tortious opening made by the ball; this opening in fact becomes nearly closed by the swelling. In such cases, free incisions should be made at the entry and exit of the ball. By introducing the finger into the opening it can be used as a guide for the incisions, which should follow the long axis of the bone. Many modern surgeons are opposed to these dilatations of fresh wounds, except for the purpose of extracting foreign substances, or for ligating an artery.

Many therapeutical methods which have undergone discredit, though really efficacious, are slow in recovering their former position. Thus it is admitted that the dilatation of all gun-shot wounds is not necessary, but it would be a great mistake to assert that they are never necessary. Of course the surgeon has to decide whether an incision should be made or not. My experience, says Stromeyer, is undoubtedly such, that in cases where a ball has pursued a long and devious track, lacerating muscles and fascia before it, a dilatation is absolutely necessary to prevent the most frightful results. For extensive suppuration will soon take place, and in order to discharge the collection of pus, many incisions will be found necessary afterwards, when they might have been prevented by an early dilatation of the original opening. This principle is also applicable to gun-shot wounds in the thigh itself. When the laceration is in the neighborhood of the larger blood vessels, then the danger increases, because the inflammation might spread to the femoral vein, and thereby cause pyæmia; for this was observed in cases where the bone itself was not injured. Besides the dilatation of the wound, there are many important precepts which should be taken into consideration to prevent the secretion of wounds from accumulating. The wounded limb should be placed in such a manner that the discharge can leave the wound by the simple laws of gravity. An opening which is too small should be dilated; also, a fistulous track should be treated in the same manner, or a counter-opening made. Isolated abscesses should be opened as soon as fluctuation is felt. Sometimes it will be found necessary to apply leeches, or cut through the fascia, to avoid a fresh swelling. Young surgeons are generally very bold in making such incisions, but they forget that their object is the discharge of pus. Instead of putting the limb in an appropriate position, in order that pus may exude from the opening, they dress the wound with charpie and sticking plaster, besides a compress and a roller, and therefore no fluid can possibly escape. When such a bandage is removed after twenty-four hours, the pus escapes in great quantity. On discovering this, these surgeons are most anxious to get rid at once of all the pus and squeeze the limb most unmercifully, to the great distress of the patient. Heedless that the pus is formed as fast as it is removed, they reäpply their bandages, and of course the pus becomes more acrid and more fetid. As usual, this fault brings on another. They apply what is called an expulsive bandage, to prevent the accumulation of pus, but really it does nothing of the kind. When this fails they resort to solutions of nitrate of silver and chloride of soda, but still the pus continues to accumulate. Let our surgeons beware of such practice as this. One good incision in the right place, will diminish the quantity of the pus, change its quality, and improve the general health of the patient. By attention to these principles we shall avoid all deposits of pus, which are otherwise inevitable.

It is important for us to notice in this place that there are two different ways in which pus may accumulate near a gun-shot wound. The most common origin of pus deposits is when it fuses beneath the cellular tissue and reaches a spot different from its origin, this percolation taking place according to the laws of gravity. In the second instance, inflammation, swelling and fluctuation, show a local tendency to the formation of pus. Here, if early incisions are made, we shall find that nothing but serum, or a gelatinous fluid will be discharged, and yet these deposits of serum are connected with larger deposits which do contain pus. This can be proved sometimes by passing the finger through the smaller cavity into the larger one. It would appear that in such cases, the fluid portions of the pus becomes infiltrated in the tissues, and by their acrid nature cause a new inflammatory process, from which, in course of time, pus originates. After a few days, when poultices are applied, pus will appear in the new incisions, which become outlets of pus from the deeper cavities. In practice, it is important to discriminate between these two different sources of pus collections. The first kind should be opened as soon as they are discovered, the last kind may require the application of leeches to prevent the formation of abscesses.

After the expulsion of all foreign substances, and the separation of fragments of bone, the inflammatory symptoms decrease, and together with it the discharge of pus. At this period of the treatment, the limb should be rolled in flannel; flannel bandages should be used in preference to cotton. Pressure is necessary to diminish the œdematous swelling of the limb; but bandages should not be applied before a fracture has been consolidated, for otherwise the moving of the limb would counterbalance any benefit derived from the bandage. When wounds, which have ceased to secrete pus, become filled with granulations, in order to accelerate the healing process, they should be dressed with pieces of soft linen or cotton corresponding with the size of the wound, dipped in a solution of nitrate of silver, of one to five grains to the ounce of water, and the whole covered with a piece of oiled silk to prevent them from drying too quickly. All cerates and salves should be dispensed with. The only dressing used after the patient leaves the bed should consist of oiled charpie.

And now, while closing these general remarks on the treatment of gun-shot wounds affecting the shaft of bones, we would again particularly call the attention of our confreres to the necessity of keeping the patients on a low diet during the inflammatory state of the wound. The diet should correspond to the antiphlogistic treatment, and consist of light soups, a few vegetables, a small quantity of bread, and a cooling beverage, which treatment sometimes has to be continued for weeks.

GUN-SHOT WOUNDS AFFECTING THE ARTICULATIONS.

Wounds affecting the larger joints are generally so dangerous as to require an early operation. Their gravity and frequency, together with their manifold varieties make them peculiarly important for the consideration of the surgeon.

DIFFERENT KINDS OF INJURIES AFFECTING THE JOINTS.

A shot by simply grazing a joint may wound only the ligaments, without causing, however, any injury to the bone itself. On the other hand, if a ball strikes the end of a bone, it may, according to its force, either go through the bone or remain in it; or it may break off a portion of it, or, finally, if it has lost its power, it may strike the epiphysis and rebound, after causing more or less damage. In such cases, where the joint is injured, the synovial capsule is not necessarily affected, but generally fissures occur, which extend through the head of the bone. The inflammation following this will sooner or late implicate the whole joint. Those wounds are the most dangerous in which the extremity of the bone, together with the synovial membrane have been torn and lacerated. The gravity of such injuries is readily understood when we remember the liability to inflammation of serous membranes in the first place, and secondly, the extent of these membranes in the joints, together with the various ligaments and tendons surrounding it, all of which will become included in the process of inflammation; besides this, the danger is increased by the destruction of the cartilaginous coverings of the bones, whereby the joint is destroyed. Moreover, the joints consisting of irregular cavities will facilitate the accumulation of the secretions of the wound, a condition which is much aggravated by the presence of splinters and other foreign substances. The extremities of bones are more spongy and vascular than other portions, consequently, when inflammation sets in, they offer a large surface for suppuration. On examining such wounds soon after the accident, the joint will be found to contain a large quantity of blood together with lymph, immediately around the spot injured by the passage of the ball. The medullary cavity itself showing the extent of the injury. As soon as suppuration begins in the wound, the extravasated blood will be decomposed, and thereby rendered offensive. This condition will extend as far as the fissures and embrace all the injured portion of bone.

PROGNOSIS OF INJURIES OF THE JOINTS.

In injuries of the larger joints, it commonly happens that serous infiltration takes place around it. Inflammation sets in, the limb begins to swell on both sides, the skin takes on a bright red color, becomes hot and tense, and the epidermis vesicated. The distal extremity of the limb becomes œdematous from obstruction of the venous circulation. Accompanying this condition, we find the following general symptoms: a frequent pulse, a dry tongue, constant thirst, and from continued suffering, the patient frequently becomes delirious. The pain is increased by the slightest motion of the limb. Suppuration soon follows, generally preceded by a chill, and pyæmia, with all its sequela closes the scene. In these cases the pus is soon decomposed and fetid; gas forms in the cavity of the joint, and the patient becomes either comatose or delirious with an icteric hue, and death rapidly follows. Such are commonly the consequences of gun-shot wounds in the knee-joint. When these symptoms appear, amputation is no longer of any avail. An early operation only, would save the life of the patient. Should a smaller joint be injured, the symptoms which we have just enumerated are usually milder in proportion, and make their appearance more slowly. For instance, if the capsule of the joint should be slightly injured and no blood penetrate into the joint, the pus may still be normal; but if the pus so formed be retained within the capsule, it will cause extensive inflammation, and finally escape by a rupture of the capsule at its weakest point. The pus will then fuse into the cellular tissue between the muscles, cause phlegmonous inflammation and the formation of abscesses. It frequently happens in such cases that pus burrows the whole extent of the limb, so that if death does not take place from pyæmia, the profuse suppuration will so endanger the life of the patient, that amputation will be the last resort.

The symptoms which set in when the synovial capsule has not been injured, are very slow and gradual, though the joint may become implicated at last from the suppuration around it. When the extremity of a bone has been struck, so as to cause fissures through the epiphysis without injury to the cartilage, the cavity of the joint in such a case may not communicate with the wound; but in the process of suppuration, the cartilages become eroded, and pus will enter the cavity of the joint, causing intense inflammation at a late day, and the patient who had been previously considered in a favorable condition, will at once present all the dangerous symptoms above enumerated.

DIAGNOSIS OF INJURIES OF THE JOINTS.

From what we have already said, it will be found difficult to ascertain, in some cases, the true extent of the injury. Doubtless, in many cases, the external appearance of the wound will be a sufficient guide in diagnosis. A wound which is considerably swollen, accompanied with much pain and high fever, with fragments of bones, and an exposed cartilage, while a bloody synovia oozes from the opening, can scarcely allow us to doubt the nature of the injury. But there are many cases, where it is very difficult to ascertain the extent of the lesion. It is well known, that a ball striking a body in an oblique manner, may glance off in a different direction, and passing beneath the skin, may come out in a distant place without penetrating the parts situated between the two openings. This has been observed in the shoulder-, elbow-, and knee-joint. But it is necessary to be cautious in concluding from a superficial examination of such a wound. For it may happen that the ball has entered the joint, while the limb was in a different position from that in which it is examined. By a change of position some muscle or tendon may obstruct the entrance of the finger, and the discharge of synovia. It is, therefore, very important to ascertain the exact position of the limb when it received the shot, and to examine it in various positions. A swelling of the capsule of the joint, though occurring imediately after the injury, is not a certain sign of the joint being affected. For this may follow any lesion in the neighborhood of the joint, and the capsule itself may be inflamed and distended without being touched by a ball.

TREATMENT OF INJURIES OF THE JOINTS.

It is well known that injuries of the joints when left alone or neglected, speedily become dangerous, they therefore, require more than all other wounds, the intervention of the surgeon. In spite of the best and most energetic treatment, the life of the patient is in jeopardy, and it therefore becomes the imperative duty of the surgeon, either to amputate the limb, or to resect the extremities of the bones, so as to simplify the wound. In some cases it may be sufficient to make a free incision into the capsule of the joint, in order to give issue to the fluids which are there abundantly secreted. But the latter treatment is accompanied with long suffering, and followed by complete ankylosis of the joint. On the other hand, the process of healing is much more rapid after a resection, and frequently some mobility may be obtained in the limb.

Wounds of the wrist and ankle will heal under favorable conditions and a proper treatment, though they entail long suffering and a stiff joint. Amputation is necessary when the bones are badly crushed. Under these circumstances a resection is not advisable; the tendons being generally implicated at the same time that it is extremely difficult to avoid the numerous vessels and nerves which surround those joints: instead of resection, it is even preferable in such cases, to make a large opening into the articulation itself.

Wounds of the larger joints call for an immediate operation, unless the capsule alone be injured, and the bones not affected. In such a case, the wound may heal by a proper antiphlogistic treatment, though it will be followed by ankylosis of the joint. As an exception, and under very favorable circumstances, it may happen that wounds in which the bones have also been implicated, heal without an operation, but the life of the patient runs a great risk, and the responsibility of the surgeon is therefore very great.

Taking all things into consideration, we should say that in cases of injuries of the larger joints, complicated with the more or less damage of the bone, it is better to amputate, although under very favorable circumstances, resection may be tried. In the olden time, when a joint was lacerated, by a ball, amputation was invariably performed.

Larrey was the first to introduce resection into military surgery. But during the revolution in Paris, of 1848, we find that the most celebrated French surgeons performed no resections. In the late war of Schleswig-Holstien, out of forty cases of complicated gun-shot wounds in the elbow-joint, in which the whole joint was resected, thirty-two were discharged

4

cured, with preservation of the limb, and only six died. It can be proved that the resection of the elbow-joint at the least, is a less dangerous operation than amputation, or disarticulation, by comparing the lists of mortality of both operations. It must be considered also, that most of these resections were made under such circumstances, that the third part of the amputated cases died. This was certainly a great triumph for conservative surgery. When we consider how helpless a man becomes after losing an arm, we can realize the advantage of preserving such a limb, although a portion of its utility be lost.

Wounds of the joints of the inferior extremities must be viewed in a different light. Thus, an artificial limb, or a wooden stump may be more servicable than a crooked or stiff leg which cannot perform its natural functions. There is still another question connected with this subject, viz : the relative gravity of the two operations, a point still undecided. Resections of the hip and knee-joint did not give good results during the war of Schleswig-Holstein ; they should, however, still be tried, and perhaps would now give better results.

GUN-SHOT WOUNDS IN DIFFERENT BONES.

UPPER EXTREMITY.

INJURIES TO THE SHAFT OF THE HUMERUS.

The liability to splinter, which is characteristic of the humerus make its injuries very dangerous. If the soft parts are much lacerated, at the same time that the shaft of the bone has been splintered, amputation is at once necessary. But when the ball has only penetrated the muscles, without injuring the vessels and nerves, an attempt should be made to preserve the arm, though the bone be considerably crushed. The chief danger of these wounds, consists in the violent inflammation which generally sets in at the inner side of the biceps. This must be combated by venesection, leeches and iced applications. If much swelling takes place, incision will be found useful. There is great difficulty in maintaining the arm in a proper position. The best way to secure it is to bandage the fore-arm across the thorax, while the wounded part of the humerus is separated from the chest by a cushion filled with oat-chaff, and covered with oiled silk ; the fractured ends of the bone are then kept together by means of Scultet's bandage. The limb is to be supported on the outside by a pasteboard splint, the whole apparatus being secured by a roller bandage passed around it and the chest. Out of twenty-five cases of complicated wounds of the shaft of the humerus, which occurred during the above mentioned war, only four died, the others recovered perfectly ; though there were several instances in which the humerus had been broken into several fragments by grape-shot. In those cases no operation whatsoever was performed, nature alone accom plishing the cure. Consolidation took place sooner or later, and a useful limb was restored to the patient.

Injuries of the bone, in the neighborhood of the elbow, may

progress favorably if the fracture be a simple one. If the humerus should be struck near its head, fissures when produced will assume a downward direction, for the head being more spongy and cellular, is not liable to such fissures. If the ball should strike the bone lower down, such fissures may go upwards and downwards. Stromeyer recommends, when these fissures are very extensive, either to amputate at once, or if amputation be not indicated, to trust to nature, and leave the wound untouched. He thinks further, that when the removal of the limb is absolutely necessary, amputation is preferable to disarticulation.

INJURIES TO THE SHOULDER-JOINT.

Gun-shot wounds of the shoulder-joint are quite frequent, and the injury may be done in every possible direction. The diagnosis of these injuries is sometimes difficult; at least to ascertain the precise extent of the injury, for the joint being covered by the whole thickness of the deltoid muscle, a thorough examination becomes almost impracticable when the deltoid is largely developed. The ball may pass through a portion of this muscle without touching the bone, or may even open the capsule of the joint, without this fact being recognized until the inflammation of the joint sets in. Fortunately, an exact diagnosis between a mere flesh wound and an injury of the capsule is not indispensable, the same antiphlogistic treatment being applicable to both injuries. They generally heal with stiffness of the joint.

When suppuration is so extensive as to endanger the life of the patient, resection of the head of the humerus is evidently indicated. Not that resection is absolutely necessary in fractures of the head of the humerus, for such wounds may heal after the splinters have been extracted, though this occurs at the expense of a stiff joint. In these cases, if resection is performed, a better result will be obtained, because some mobility generally follows. This operation may be performed at once or after suppuration has taken place.

The resection of this joint, says Esmarch, has given us such good results and so rapidly, that if we add to this the benefit of an artificial joint instead of an ankylosed limb, we can not hesitate to declare that *resection should be performed at once in all injuries of the shoulder-joint, in which the head of the humerus is fractured from gun-shot wounds.*

The rule which we have just given is based upon the following statistics: eight cases were left to the curative efforts of nature; of these five died, and in one it was yet undecided after six months' treatment whether an operation would not still be required. Out of nineteen cases, where resection of the head of the humerus was performed, only seven died, and twelve recovered perfectly, with a more or less useful limb. In none of these cases did ankylosis take place. Some were healed in less than three months. Among those cases which proved fatal, some had been operated during the inflammatory stage, others were treated in unhealthy places, where the simplest wounds gave rise to pyæmia.

Larrey and Guthrie have established the rule, that resection should only be performed in those cases where only the head of the humerus is injured; but if the injury extends as far as the medulla, the limb should be taken off at the joint.

The statements of Stromeyer and Esmarch are opposed to this. During the Schleswig-Holstein campaign, most of the resections included a portion of the shaft of the bone, sometimes as much as four and five inches. If the ball, after fracturing the head of the humerus, should have entered the chest, it may still be advisable to operate, provided there is a chance of saving the patient's life; the resulting loss of blood would be more serviceable than otherwise.

We shall now give those methods of resection which we think the best.

Method of Langenbeck.—A longitudinal incision is made in front of the joint, beginning at the anterior edge of the acromion, extending from two to four inches in the direction of the tendon of the long head of the biceps, which is reached after the skin and deltoid muscle have been divided. The sheath of the tendon should now be opened on its outside, the knife being passed closely to the inner edge of the greater tuberosity of the humerus; after the tendon has been exposed, it can be recognized by its silvery hue; the knife should then be introduced into the joint, the point being carried forward and the back resting against the bone. The capsule being opened, the cartilage of the head will be seen beneath the anterior edge of the acromion. The tendon of the biceps should now be taken out of the bicipital groove by means of a blunt hook, drawn inwards and held by an assistant (the edges of the wound during this time being separated by hooks). The assistant who holds the arm should now rotate the limb inwards, by which the larger tuberosity comes into view. A circular incision should then be directed around this tuberosity, beginning at the opening of the capsule, and ending at the external edge of the bicipital groove, the convexity of the cut being outwards. By this incision, the tendon of the supraspinatus, infraspinatus and teres major will be divided. The arm is now rotated outwards, in order to bring the lesser tuberosity in front, and the tendon of the biceps should be replaced in the groove. A semi-lunar incision will then be carried around the lesser tuberosity, by which the tendon of the subscapularis muscle is divided. By means of these incisions, which have the form of the Greek letter Φ, the capsule, together with all the tendons and ligaments, will be divided down to the bone; so that the head of the humerus can now be pushed out, the tendon of the biceps being again drawn inwards by means of a hook. The head of the bone should be pushed out of its socket and made to project out of the wound, at which time the operator introduces a blunt-pointed knife behind the head of the bone, dividing the posterior part of the capsule and separating the pectoralis major, latissimus, dorsi and teres major as low down as the saw must be applied. This is done by carrying the elbow backwards and upwards, so that the upper end of the humerus projects out of the wound. After the head of the bone has been removed, the arm should be bandaged in the manner above described, the greater part of the incision being brought together by sutures.

This method is of easy execution, when the head of the humerus is not completely separated from the bone by the force of the ball; but if this should be the case, then another incision, two inches long, should meet the upper part of the first incision at right angles, cutting across a portion of the deltoid muscle near the acromion. By this means a sufficient space will be had to remove the head of the bone or its fragments. The objections to this method is the difficulty of obtaining of a free discharge of the secreted fluids from the wound.

Method of Stromeyer.—The following method was proposed by Stromeyer and performed with the best results. A semi-lunar cut beginning at the posterior edge of the acromion, should be directed downwards three inches towards the outer side of the humerus, the convexity of this incision being outward. In this manner the joint will be opened from above and behind. The arm should then be drawn forwards and upwards, thereby exposing the anterior portion of the capsule together with the tendons and ligaments, all of which should be divided with the exception of the long tendon of the biceps. By this method, the secretions of the wound are easily discharged while the patient lies on his back. No infiltration of pus can occur, and the results have proved the excellence of the process. Patients have recovered in half the time required by the other methods, where the secretions are not so easily removed. The greater part of the incision should be sewed up, and only a portion left open for the drainage of the wound. The arm should be flexed at right angles and bandaged to the body. The wound itself should be dressed with cold water applications. When suppuration takes place and the pus looks healthy, warm water dressings may be substituted, and finally it may be covered with oiled charpie. The cavity will soon fill up with granulations. The arm should not be moved during the suppurative stage. The wound can be syringed with warm water to keep it clean. When the wound begins to cicatrize, the limb should be moved gently and gradually until mobility is established.

As we have already stated, out of nineteen resections of the shoulder joint, made during the three years' campaign in Schleswig-Holstein, seven cases only died, all of which succumbed from pyæmia. The post-mortem examination of all these cases revealed either the decomposition of the medullary portion of the bone, or phlebitis of the axillary vein, and sometimes both together.

The length of time which intervened, says Esmarch, between the wound and the operation, seemed to exercise some influence upon the result; thus out of six cases operated upon in the first twenty-four hours after the injury, two died. In three cases, resection was performed while inflammation was at its height, on the third and fourth days; of these, two proved fatal. Secondary resections were performed in ten cases after suppuration had existed for some time; of these, three died. Some of the latter, however, would have been saved, had the operation been performed earlier, say in the first twenty-four hours. We should therefore state the rule, either to operate at once, or postpone it until suppuration has been fully established. During this time the antiphlogistic treatment will prepare them for the subsequent operation. Another remarkable result observed in those resections was that the mortality from resection of the left arm was greater, as compared to that of the right arm, an observation which was also made in resections of the elbow.

INJURIES OF THE ELBOW.

Gun-shot wounds of the elbow are comparatively more dangerous than those of the shoulder. Instances where recovery took place after serious injuries of the bones, are very rare. It is therefore laid down as a rule in military surgery, in all cases where the joint is implicated, that the limb must be sacrificed in order to save the life of the patient. But in later times, resections of the elbow-joint have been performed where amputation would have taken place previously. Langenbeck and Stromeyer are entitled to the credit of establishing this conquest of conservative surgery. Larrey never performed it, Guthrie mentioned it but never executed it himself, and the military reports up to the year of 1848–9 show that this operation had not been performed during the revolutionary epoch in Paris or Italy, in Berlin or Hungary. During the war of Schleswig-Holstein, the principal injuries which occurred to the elbwow-joint were as follows: In most cases the ball had struck the ulna, while the soldier was either loading or firing his gun, the arm being in a bent position. Sometimes the ball entered the soft parts of the forearm, went some distance along the muscles, crushing the radius or ulna. In very few cases the condyles of the humerus were injured, a fact which can only be explained by the position of the humerus, being protected by the radius and ulna when the arm is flexed on the forearm.

"In all cases, says Stromeyer, when I diagnosed an injury of the bones of the elbow, I did not hesitate to perform resection at once. The joint was opened from behind by an incision at the inner side of the olecranon. A second incision was then made perpendicular to the first, opening the joint from the head of the radius to the *external* condyle. This incision should extend over the olecranon and divide the tendon of the triceps. After the joint has been opened on the posterior portion, exposing fully the articulation, all the loose fragments of bone should be extracted; even those which are still in connection should be taken out with the knife or bone forceps, the ulnar nerve being, however, carefully respected. If the ulna was alone injured, the end of it should be sawed off, with a corresponding portion of the radius. Of the latter, however, no more than the head and neck should be taken off, though the fissures of the other bone, the ulna, might have extended further down. In such cases to have removed all the injured portions of the bone, would have caused the sacrifice of three or four inches, an operation which would be more complicated and less advantageous; for, even if the patient recovered and the limb was preserved, we should not have had either an artificial joint or ankylosis. I have never had cause to regret having acted in this cautious manner, but on the contrary, have observed that a new bone was established from that part of the ulna, which otherwise would have been sacrificed. When the radius was fractured below the neck, the fragments were extracted, the ends being smoothed off with a saw. In such a case the olcranon alone was removed from the adjoining bone, as this would otherwise project after the healing of the wound, and cause much annoyance."

The ulna being the bone upon which the solidity of the joint chiefly depends, it should be preserved as much as possible. After removing the fractured portions from the ulna and radius, and sawing the ends of these bones, it may be necessary to saw off likewise a portion of the trochlea humeri. In many cases the bone need not be touched at all, it being sufficient to pare off the cartilage with the knife; a process which did not interfere with the healing of the wound.

When the adjoining part of the humerus is also injured, the operation is somewhat difficult. Generally one of the two condyles will be crushed, and the fissure extends beyond the capsular ligament. To resect in such a case, all the fissured portion, would involve a loss of some two and a half inches of bone. It is, in fact, only necessary to resect a small portion of the injured bone, but then the olecranon process of the ulna must be removed at the same time. In dressing the wound, the upper portion should be brought together by means of sutures, and the lower portion left open for the discharge of the secretions.

The statistics of this operation are exceedingly favorable. Whilst under the same circumstances most of the amputated cases died, most of the resected cased recovered perfectly and retained the mobility of the hand, though there was generally partial ankylosis of the elbow.

There are, undoubtedly, cases where amputation instead of resection must be performed. For instance, when the ball, besides shattering the bone, has likewise torn the main vessels at the inner side of the arm, causing bloody infiltration of the forearm and secondary hemorrhage, then the brachial artery must necessarily be tied, and this would cause mortification of the forearm, as the collateral vessels which usually keep up the circulation could scarcely be avoided in performing resection of the joint. Amputation is furthermore indicated when the soft parts around the joint are extensively lacerated.

We find the following statistical results obtained during the campaign of Schleswig-Holstein: out of fifty-four cases of amputation of the humerus, nineteen died; out of forty cases of resections of the elbow, only six died. On the other hand, the wound after resection heals more slowly than after amputation; but when we consider that the limb is preserved, the advantage of the two operations can scarcely be weighed in the same balance. It is a strange fact that the healing process is much shorter, the more we have to sacrifice of the ligaments and capsule of the joint.

As to the treatment of a resected joint, rest and a comfortable position are the main objects to be attended to. Immediately after the operation, the limb should be placed on a wooden concave splint, padded with cotton wadding, covered with oiled silk, to prevent it from being soiled. The splint should reach from the upper third of the humerus downwards to the ends of the fingers, and should be bent at the elbow at an angle of 140°; care being taken at the same time, that no undue pressure be exercised on the internal condyles. For this purpose an opening should be made into the splint. The arm resting in this way on the excavated splint should be placed on a large cushion filled with chopped straw and fastened in this position. The wound itself must be dressed with cold water applications, and when suppuration is established, with warm water. When the suppuration ceases, oiled charpie should be used to cover the wound.

It is of the utmost importance that the arm be moved from the splint. A sufficient quantity of charpie should be stuffed on both sides of the arm, in order to absorb the secretions of the wound. This can be replaced when soiled, without moving the arm. If pus collects in the tissues, it is not proper to press or syringe the wound, it being preferable to remove the pus by a new incision. After the wound has progressed so far as to become filled by granulations, the limb may be cautiously raised and bandaged with flannel. At this period warm water baths of the whole arm will prove very serviceable, to reëstablish the mobility of hand and fingers.

It is a well known fact, that artificial joints, can only be produced by motion; it is, therefore, important to make an early attempt to establish the joint. We may begin to move the arm cautiously before the wound has completely closed. But if this should irritate the wound, giving the granulations a livid appearance, we should stop the manipulations; for otherwise inflammation and hæmorrhage might ensue. As soon as the wound has completely healed, we must advise the patient to move his arm frequently; but this being painful and therefore commonly neglected by the patient, it must be done by the nurse or some other attendant. When ankylosis takes place, it is generally to be attributed to negligence in this respect. The importance of these precepts in regard to the after-treatment, says Esmarch, was clearly proved in those cases which happened to fall into the hands of the Danes, after resection had been performed. The Danish surgeons never performed this operation, and therefore had no idea of the importance of motion to the resected limb. When those prisoners were exchanged, they therefore returned with ankylosed joints. It was observed also that the ankylosed limbs were bent at an angle of 130° to 140°, which was the position when the arm was treated. This degree of flexion was chosen because it seemed to give the patient less pain than any other position, and in case of partial ankylosis rendered the limb more useful.

It has been observed that mobility of the joint is not dependant upon the extent of resected surface; for it happened that in some cases ankylosis took place where a large portion of the bones was removed, while others recovered with a comparatively useful limb, though a small portion of the bone had been taken off.

INJURIES OF THE FOREARM.

An injury of one or both bones of the forearm, from a gun-shot, seldom requires amputation when there are no complications to endanger the life of the patient. Extensive inflammation of both bones may be controlled by leeching and cold applications. The treatment of such cases is simple: the forearm should be placed on a splint, extending from the elbow to the end of the fingers. All tight bandages should be carefully avoided. In the beginning, iced applications should be made; and afterwards, warm fomentations. The splinters must be extracted when detached by the suppurative process. At a later period, flannel bandages are of a great benefit. Forty cases of injuries of the forearm are reported. In six of these both bones were fractured; in sixteen cases the radius, and in eighteen cases the ulna alone were injured. All recovered.

INJURIES OF THE WRIST.

Gun-shot wounds of the wrist are very dangerous on account of the inflammation which generally follows such injuries. They frequently affect the whole system, and show a great tendency to pyæmia. This can be explained by the numerous tendons which cover this joint, retained in their positions by the annular ligament. When inflammation is developed in this region, pus collects beneath these ligaments, causing pressures on the nerves and producing intense pain. Moreover, suppuration of the medullary portion of the bone generally takes place, embracing the chances of pyæmia, and then amputation itself is of no avail. When the swelling is not very extensive, an energetic antiphlogistic treatment must be adopted; iced applications, leeches, and even venesection, together with small doses of opium must be resorted to. Incisions may be made to relieve the swelling and pain. If the soft parts around the wrist are much lacerated, an early amputation is required.

INJURIES OF THE HAND.

Injuries of the second series of the carpi and metacarpi, together with the phalanges, are not so dangerous as injuries of the first row of bones of the hand, and do not absolutely require an operation. The expectant method should be followed here. No operation at least is justified when the wounded were not treated immediately after the injury. Suppuration sets in at an early period, and as long as the acute stage continues, the surgeon should not interfere with the wound.

Wounds of the fingers occur very frequently in battle. When disarticulation or amputation are performed at an early day, no serious symptoms are found to rise. But it was observed during the late campaign of Schleswig-Holstein, that all operations performed upon the fingers forty-eight hours after the injury occurred, only increased the inflammation, caused suppuration in the course of the tendons, and occasioned stiffness of one or more fingers, if not the whole hand. During the campaign, says Stromeyer, I never performed disarticulation of a finger, except immediately after the injury was received. I have never observed tetanus supervene after these wounds. The beneficial effects of venesection are abundantly proved by many instances.

All injuries of the hand should be treated by placing the extremity on a board adapted for that purpose. Poultices are useful when suppuration has commenced, and more so than in all other wounds of the upper extremities; they also will be required for a longer period.

LOWER EXTREMITY.

INJURIES TO THE SHAFT OF THE FEMUR.

The simplest and least dangerous accident that can happen this bone from a gun-shot wound, is, that the ball should fracture the bone without much crushing or splintering. An accurate examination of these wounds is often difficult, especially when the limb is already much swollen. If the bone be fractured by a large projectile, and the soft parts extensively lacerated, then all idea of preserving the limb should be abandoned, and the sooner amputation is performed the better for the patient. The gravity of the injury increases in proportion as the wound is nearer the trunk; inflammation, suppuration and phlebitis being more likely to occur in a short and moveable fragment, than in a longer one. Instead of the plastic exudation which takes place around the ends of bone in simple fractures, in these cases the fragments are exposed to suppuration, followed by necrosis; so that the possibility of union by the formation of callus is destroyed. The provisional callus is sometimes formed, however, around the necrosed fragments, and partial consolidation takes place. Then the suppuration diminishes though it will not disappear until the sequestra are expelled. When left to the slow efforts of nature, this may require years for its completion. All these reasons should decide the military surgeon in favor of immediate amputation, at least in the great majority of such cases. Such, at all events is the present state of military surgery. Nevertheless, the question arises whether it would not be proper to attempt to save the limb under favorable circumstances. Experience has proved that this can only be done when the treatment is commenced at once, without any transportation of the patient. No bandage however carefully adjusted, can obviate the injury caused by transportation; and when we take into consideration the rude wagons commonly used to convey the wounded, it becomes evident no subsequent care could neutralize the damage so caused. It is much better to convey such wounded patients to some house near the battle-field, and incur the risk of falling into the enemy's hands, than to transport them. The dictates of humanity, the precepts of science, command that such cases should be sacred alike to friend and foe. If, therefore, the surgeon expects or undertakes to save the limb, the first care is to place it in a proper position. Unless the swelling be already too extensive, the fractured ends of bone should be adjusted, while the patient is under the influence of chloroform. Long cushions filled with oat-chaff should be placed on both sides of the limb, and extension maintained by wooden splints resting on these, this being secured by some appropriate bandage. The whole apparatus should be so disposed, that an easy access to the wound can be had. A strict antiphlogistic treatment is absolutely required. All probing and otherwise irritating the wound under pretence of searching for foreign bodies, should not be practiced. The wound should be dressed with care and delicacy, and it is quite unsurgical to press the wound or raise the limb. As soon as the inflammatory stage has gone by, Scultet's bandage can be used with good advantage and the splints applied more closely. In case the patient suffers from the limb being placed in a straight position, a double inclined plane will be found very useful. Of course the surgeon should endeavor, as much as possible, to retain the normal length of the limb. But when suppuration is too profuse and long continued, threatening the life of the patient, then, says Stromeyer, it is well enough to save the limb, even at the expense of some shortening. By allowing the muscles to contract naturally, the healthy portions of bone will overlap each other, and becoming readily united, suppuration will soon cease. This distinguished author says, that within eight days, he has observed the most decided advantage following this plan of treatment. In such cases, the limb should be placed on a double inclined plane, great care being taken to maintain it in its proper position by means of the foot-board.

The great trochanter is sometimes splintered without a complete fracture of the femur, an accident which is sometimes very dangerous on account of the spongy nature of this part of the bone. An antiphlogistic treatment should be instituted, and free incision be made when it is necessary to get rid of the pus. It is dangerous to attempt to remove splinters at an early period, for it is well known that access of air, which is thereby occasioned, is very prejudicial to the wound, generally causing suppuration and inflammation of the joint.

INJURIES OF THE HIP JOINT.

Gun-shot wounds of the hip-joint are almost always fatal, partly on account of the complications which generally exist, and partly on account of the tendency of such wounds to pyæmia. Fortunately this injury seldom occurs. Larrey, who undoubtedly had the greatest experience of any military surgeon up to the present time, says in his surgical clinick, that he never saw a case of the kind. This can be explained by the fact that a wound affecting the hip-joint generally extends to the contents of the pelvis, and therefore proves rapidly fatal; moreover, post-mortem examinations are seldom made after important battles, and no means exist of ascertaining the proportion of the different wounds.

The diagnosis of these injuries is difficult, from the fact of their being deeply situated and covered by several thick and powerful muscles, interfering with an accurate examination. The great swelling which rapidly takes place, the acute pain occasioned by motion of the limb, are the only symptoms which can lead us to infer, that the joint is implicated.

Injuries of the neck of the bone, or in the neighborhood of the great trochanter, are not so rare, though quite as difficult to diagnose as injuries of the joint. The characteristic symptoms of fracture of the neck are not apparent at first. Several such cases have been observed that were not recognized before the symptoms of pyæmia set in. Without surgical intervention such cases ended fatally, on account of the fissures which generally extended to the head of the femur, so that when suppuration took place, pus was transmitted to the capsule of the joint, causing inflammation of the hip-joint and all its sequela.

When the trochanters are injured, they are predisposed to suppuration on account of their spongy nature, and this soon extends to the medullary portion of the bone, whence pus will be taken up by the veins and carried throughout the system. Surgical intervention being necessary, the choice is between disarticulation or resection. During the war of Schleswig-Holstein, disarticulation of the femur was performed seven times, five of which were by Langenbeck; of these one survived, a young man aged seventeen years. This unfortunate result induced Stromeyer to try resection in the following case, which we relate as highly instructive.

At the battle of Kolding, on the 23d of April, 1849; a Danish musketeer received a ball which fractured the left femur, passing in an oblique direction through both trochanters. The local and general symptoms appeared so favorable at first, that it was thought likely to heal without any operation. The patient was placed in a proper position and treated on the antiphlogistic plan. Nevertheless, extensive suppuration took place, the pus becoming decomposed and offensive. An incision was made through the wound, to allow the free discharge of pus, and to remove any splinters that might be detached. This incision extended upwards, four inches above the gun-shot wound, and the same distance below it; a few terse fragments were then extracted. On further examination it was found that a fissure extended through the neck of the femur, extending to the capsule ; the upper portion of the fractured bone was then seized by means of a strong hooked forceps, and the capsule and ligamentum teres were cut with a scalpel, so that the head of the bone was thus disarticulated. The lower end of the femur was next pushed out of the wound, and all the injured portion, two inches long, sawed off below the lesser trochanter. The operation was not a difficult one, and the condition of the patient improved during the first two days after the operation. There was less fever, and some hope was entertained of saving the life of the patient. Nevertheless, on the third day a chill announced the dreaded symptoms of purulent absorption ; a secondary abscess was formed on the right shoulder, and in the foot ; the patient died on the 20th of May. At the post-mortem examination, it was found that the tuberosity of the ischium was injured, and that the medullary portion of that bone was infiltrated with decomposed pus. The foot and shoulder-joints on the right side were also filled with pus.

There is no doubt that resection is a less dangerous operation than disarticulation. We would, therefore, advise resection as a preferable operation in all cases, where no laceration of the anterior side of the femur has taken place, the vessels and nerves being at the same time uninjured. The best time for this operation is after the suppurative process has commenced, for by this means we give him all the chances of life and lessen the dangers of pyæmia.

INJURIES OF THE KNEE-JOINT.

The dangers which we have already stated as usually accompanying injuries of the joints, reach their maximum in those of the knee-joint. The injury may be situated in the synovial capsule alone, or it may implicate the bone likewise. The former kind are rare, and yet the inflammation and suppuration which follow, generally require amputation of the thigh at a later period, though much could be done by an antiphlogistic treatment to diminish the inflammation and allow the wound to heal. There are few cases on record who have recovered under this method. It must be borne in mind, that though the wound may heal externally, and consequently no synovia be discharged, still chronic inflammation of the synovial membrane may exist, causing the wound to reöpen, so that an amputation of the thigh will become necessary. The fear of ankylosis should not therefore prompt us to attempt too early a motion of the limb. Most of the injuries of the knee-joint implicate the bones more or less. It is important, though difficult, to make a diagnosis of the extent and seat of injury. When the bones are extensively fractured, the intense swelling and pain of the knee-joint will hardly allow a mistake on the subject, though the finger cannot reach the full extent of the wound.

We would therefore formulate the following proposition: *All gun-shot wounds of the knee-joint in which the condyles of the femur or tibia are injured require immediate amputation of the thigh.* This sad truth, long stated by the old authorities, is unfortunately still true at the present time. Esmarch says, that, regretting to sacrifice a limb for an apparently trifling wound, he was often prompted by pity to attempt its preservation, but as often did he repent the trial. The symptoms of purulent infection set in so quickly that medical intervention proved of no avail; and even when a powerful antiphlogistic treatment diminished inflammation, and apparently gave hope of a favorable prognosis, yet amputation had to be performed at a later period, and then with little chance of preserving the patient's life. This statement is fully confirmed by Guthrie, in his treatise of gun-shot wounds of the extremities. He says, that wounds of the knee-joint, when one or both epiphyses are fractured, require immediate amputation: he states that he never saw a case recover without it, and that if there is only a slight injury of the patella, the cure may be tried without amputation, but not so if the synovial capsule has been touched. For though the wound will probably heal, amputation will become necessary at a later period. He recommends an active antiphlogistic treatment as absolutely necessary, and deprecates warm poultices as the infallible precursors of amputation.

During the campaign of Schleswig-Holstein, the results of amputation of the thigh were so unfavorable, that it was always reluctantly performed. Out of one hundred and twenty-eight cases, seventy-seven died, and only fifty-one recovered. Many of the cases which proved fatal had been amputated after infiltration and suppuration had already taken place.

If the shaft of the femur or tibia has been struck some distance from the joint, it is at times impossible to say whether the joint be implicated or not. In younger individuals at least, hope may be entertained that fissures have not progressed so far as the head of the bone; such cases recover without any inflammation or stiffness of the joint.

INJURIES OF THE LEG.

Although one or both bones of the leg may be injured, the limb should be preserved, unless hemorrhage or other complications make amputation necessary. A ball may pass through the head of the tibia without splintering the bone. If the ball should be lodged in this part of the tibia it should be extracted, either by enlarging the opening or by means of the gouge. If the tibia be struck at its middle or lower portion, the ball passing through, the bone is generally much splintered. In these cases extensive suppuration is apt to follow, and therefore the danger of purulent absorbtion will influence our prognosis. In the campaign of Schleswig-Holstein a partial resection of the tibia for the purpose of removing the splinters, was scarcely better than the expectant treatment, and commonly resulted in pyæmia. Stromeyer says that in those cases where the tibia was much damaged, he preferred to amputate, even though the fibula was not injured. He states further, that having frequently seen pyæmia follow amputation likewise, he does not feel authorized to pass a final judgment on the subject. It must be taken into consideration also, that many of those cases did not come under his care until twenty-four hours after the accident. It is evident that where the circumstances of the amputation would be more favorable, the results would be correspondingly modified.

We need scarcely say, that when both bones of a leg are crushed, amputation will generally be required.

If the fibula only be injured, the wound need not be considered dangerous, and nature will generally remove the splinters.

The apparatus for the treatment of gun-shot wounds of the leg, consists of the fracture box we have already described ; into this the limb should be placed when both bones are fractured : a paste-board splint will be sufficient when the fibula alone is injured.

When the malleoli are struck by grazing shots, amputation will not be required, though such wounds generally heal with ankylosis of the tibio-tarsal articulation. Should the lower end of the tibia be much crushed by a ball, amputation is certainly indicated.

INJURIES OF THE FOOT.

The most dangerous wounds of the foot are caused by bombshells. Stromeyer says, that they frequently become gangrenous, followed by prostration of the system, and sometimes tetanus. Injuries from musket-balls are not so dangerous, and under favorable circumstances generally recover. The treatment consists of iced applications, leeches, and saline purgatives, otherwise, the same treatment may applied as that described, for injuries of the hand.

GUN-SHOT WOUNDS OF THE BODY.

Injuries affecting the head and trunk seldom require surgical methods, other than the general antiphlogistic treatment.

In gun-shot wounds of the *lower maxillary bone*, no splinters should be removed except those which are entirely loose, leaving the other fragments to be afterwards separated by the suppurative process. It will be observed that in most cases of injuries of the lower maxillary, however extensive they may be, union will take place after the removal of a large portion of the bone by the suppurative process; for the periosteum being retained, a new formation of bone will take place. Resection, therefore, may be considered bad surgery. Bandaging is also unnecessary; the chief care consists in keeping the mouth clean, which can be done by syringing it with cold and later with warm water. This is important in order to obviate the irritative properties of pus, which when swallowed, cause disorder of the stomach and bowels.

The *clavicule* more than any other bone, demonstrates the advantage of the expectant method of treatment: there any operation, whatsoever, at the begining is useless, if not dangerous.

Injuries of the *scapula* only prove fatal, if the fracture extends to the joint. In such cases, the wound never should be dilated, and no fragments ought to be extracted until it has been ascertained that the joint is not implicated.

CONCLUSION.

Our task is finished. We have prepared it with the zeal which a good cause deserves, and we now send it forth on its own merits. The rules which we have laid down in the foregoing pages, are derived from the experience gathered in the campaign of Schleswig-Holstein. Though some surgical reports of the late war in the Crimea, and Italy, are sometimes at variance with these precepts, we think, nevertheless, they will stand the test of time and true science.

And now, Confrères, Surgeons of the army of the South! we have dedicated this pamphlet to you, and sincerely trust that it may be a safe guide on the battle-field; in the ambulance, and in the hospital. Should it be the means of saving one human life, or, even one useful limb, our labor will not have been in vain.

M. SCHUPPERT.

Norman Publishing is a division of Jeremy Norman & Company, Inc., leading international dealers in rare books and manuscripts in the history of medicine and science.

The following people collaborated on the production of *Notes and Observatons on Army Surgery* and *A Treatise on Gun-Shot Wounds*

Diana Hook, Associate Editor
Steven Hiatt, Copy Editor
Jill Rotenberg, Project Manager
Martha Steele, Editorial Assistant
Seventeenth Street Studios, Designer

The layout was done by Donna Kelley at Zetatype Desktop Publishers of San Francisco, using Ventura Publisher. The type is Bodoni, a Postscript font from Adobe Systems.

Linotronic output by Pinnacle Type, San Francisco.

Printed and bound by Braun-Brumfield, Inc., Ann Arbor.

With its geometrical framework, the Norman Publishing logo resembles the constructed letters of the Renaissance, but there the resemblance ends. The logo incorporates the capital letter N within an arc of the logarithmic spiral, one of the most beautiful mathematical curves appearing in nature. It links together the graphic arts and the sciences, reflecting the dual commitments of Norman Publishing.

NORMAN
PUBLISHING TM